The Story of Cardiology in Newcastle

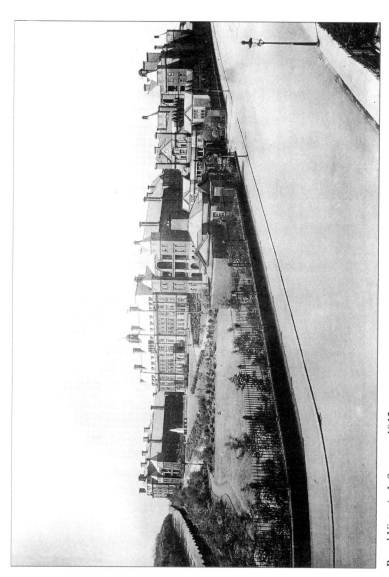

Royal Victoria Infirmary, 1912

The Story of Cardiology in Newcastle

Hewan Dewar

Durham Academic Press

First published in 1998 by
Durham Academic Press
1 Hutton Close
South Church
Bishop Auckland
Durham

ISBN 1-900838-079

Typeset by Carnegie Publishing, 18 Maynard St, Preston
Printed and bound by Antony Rowe Ltd, Chippenham

To my wife, Margaret,
and to our children,
John and Caroline

CONTENTS

Authors of Chapters

Chapter 1., H.A. Dewar with contribution from D.G. Julian
Chapters 2., 5., 8. & 9., H.A. Dewar
Chapter 3. & 6., R.G. Gold
Chapter 4., H.A. Dewar and A.S. Hunter
Chapter 7., Part I) H.A. Dewar; Part II) G. Terry

ILLUSTRATIONS

ACKNOWLEDGEMENTS

I wish to thank the following for photographs:

Mr G. W. Falcon (Newc. Gen. Hosp.), Professor F. T. Farmer (Marion Farmer), Dr D. Girling (Ary Blesovsky), Dr J. Griffin (Selwyn Griffin), Mrs R. Jacobson (Lionel Jacobson), Newcastle City Libraries Information Service (R.V.I. in 1912), Sally Odd (R.V.I. and Freeman Hospital in 1997) and Dr M. Szekely (Paul Szekely), and also those who kindly provided photographs of themselves. I am grateful to Dr Keith Evemy for lending me the Minutes of the Newcastle Cardiac Club, and to Dr Gordon Terry for the account of the Northern Region Cardiology Group.

The following were very helpful, when I interviewed them for information on Cardiology in Newcastle, both before and after the piece contributed to 'Medicine in Northumbria', namely Dr P. C. Adams, Mr A. Hedley Brown, Mrs P. Burns S.R.N., Professor R. W. F. Campbell, Mr R. Dobson, Dr S. S. Furniss, Mr S. G. Griffin (dec. since), Dr C. B. Henderson (dec. since), Dr F. S. Jackson, Dr D. S. Reid, Mrs Anne Townsend S.R.N.

Professor Heather Ashton kindly gave permission for Mrs. Margaret Cheek to type some considerable parts of the text.

Foreword

This book, for which Hewan Dewar has asked me to write a foreword, brings back vivid memories of my early childhood in Newcastle. I am very touched by the numerous references to my father. In those childhood years after the First World War, my father was developing his private practice and, at the same time, displaying in both hospital and medical school, those qualities of compassionate care, lucid instruction and wisdom, which the author so much admired. Our home in Ellison Place was geared to that private practice. Although my father's private secretary, Mr. George Dillingham, who had served as his batman in the war and remained with him throughout his professional life, was most efficient, crises would arise. When they did – as for example is described in the book when some electrographic tracings had to be developed in a hurry – my mother and any of the rest of the family would step in to help. Although I left home at the age of eighteen, I have retained great affection for and interest in Newcastle. I return to it as occasion arises with the greatest of pleasure.

I am not, of course, qualified to understand the technical advances which have been made in both the diagnosis and treatment of heart disease, and am appreciative of the efforts made in this book to render them comprehensible to the layman. It is reassuring to learn how some of those advances, especially those made most recently, have made those techniques both more effective and less daunting to the patient.

I am happy to know that my native city has contributed, and is still contributing so much, to the medical speciality which, apart from his family, was my father's most absorbing interest.

Basil Hume
Archbishop of Westminster

INTRODUCTION

This account of the development of the study of heart disease in Newcastle upon Tyne began in 1991, when Professor David Gardner-Medwin was preparing to host next year in the city a meeting of the Medical History Section of the Royal Society of Medicine. For that meeting he compiled a book entitled *Medicine in Northumbria*. I contributed to it a small chapter called 'Cardiology in Newcastle – the first 60 years'. It covered the period 1908 to 1968. Later I decided to bring that account up to date, and am glad to acknowledge here the permission of Professor Gardner-Medwin, representing the Pybus Society, to reproduce most of that text in this update.

Since I had retired from my post as Physician and Cardiologist at the Royal Victoria Infirmary (R.V.I.) in 1978, I asked a number of former colleagues, younger than me, to help in the task. In most instances this has enabled me to take responsibility for the whole text. In the first chapter, the bulk of it written by me, I am indebted to Professor Julian for an account of the origin and development of the new University Department of Cardiology, of which he was the first head. In the case of Paediatrics, Dr Stewart Hunter has kindly supplied the later part of the actual text. For the Surgical section, Dr Ronald Gold has skilfully incorporated information from *Medicine in Northumbria* into the text, and added so much more from his personal knowledge that the chapter is essentially his alone. The chapter on Cardiac Pacing is totally his.

Before writing the early account, published in *Medicine in Northumbria*, I interviewed a large number of people, some, alas, no longer living. For the updating I must thank a number of others, who gave me, either by letter or personally, a great deal of valuable information. Professor R. W. F. Campbell was particularly helpful. Above all I am grateful to Dr R. G. Gold, who has not only written two chapters, but also supplied information, advice and criticism, and also a few scattered pieces of text in other places. Finally I am especially delighted that Cardinal Basil Hume has written a foreword to this story of Cardiology in Newcastle, which in its early years owed everything to the enthusiasm and farsightedness of his father.

In writing this extended account, two important decisions had to be made. One was whether to make it intelligible and reasonably appealing to the general public as well as to my profession. The original chapter in *Medicine in Northumbria* had been exclusively addressed to the latter, but the general public is nowadays so liberally nourished by both the B.B.C. and I.T.V. on medical programmes, that technical terms do not baffle them in the way they would have done in the early days of this narrative. However a glossary of some of the medical terms is provided. There is also much interest in local history, including medical history. The story, therefore, has been purposely phrased so as to be, in large part at least, intelligible to others than doctors, and I can only hope that the latter will not find it too 'popularised'. Whether the public will find it interesting is another matter.

The second decision to be made was whether to include the names of persons still alive. Anxieties on this point had been raised in my mind by the comment made to me by Professor Sir William Hume about the (excellent) short *History of the Royal Victoria Infirmary* which he wrote in 1951 as part of that Institution's bi-centenary celebrations. He had, he said, deliberately mentioned only the dead, so that no-one could complain that he had been left out! But the high standing of Newcastle's cardiology today owes most to those still practising it. Not to make that clear would inflict much injustice. If a patient has a troublesome disorder of the rhythm of the heart or has been born with a defect in it, there is to-day nowhere in the world where it would be dealt with more efficiently than in Newcastle. There is also the thought that I am now a good 10 years older than Professor Hume was when he made that self-denying decision, and when one reaches a certain age, accusations of partiality and of vanity are rarely levelled with much force in case they prove to be medically dangerous!

As an example of the problem, a list of all the research papers published on cardiological subjects from Newcastle in the nearly two decades since I retired would, I fear, make very arduous reading. To make a selection is an invidious task, which I could not face. With cowardice I have therefore broadly indicated the principal areas in which research has been directed and have provided, with Professor Campbell's permission, some of the lists of the staffing of the Freeman Hospital, which he has sent each year to the British Heart Foundation. It includes all consultants in cardiology, whether part of the Academic Unit or not, together with the names of most of the research workers who held B.H.F. grants. I fear that it may not include all of the latter nor the names of some whose research was funded otherwise or did not need money at all. To them I can only offer my apologies. I would, however, make the point that, since about the time I retired, tracking down research references has been enormously facilitated by the introduction of Medline. In the early part of this narrative, if neither names nor references had been given, identification would have involved extremely tedious searches through volume after volume of *Index Medicus*. Fortunately Professor Campbell's secretary also holds a list of all the research papers which have been published since the Academic Unit was set up by Professor Julian in 1975.

Meanwhile it seems helpful to paint in a little of the medical background. To those not familiar with the City of Newcastle, one should perhaps explain that the Medical School began in a tentative way in 1832, but achieved a formal status in 1883, when a rather charming red brick building, now the Faculty of Law of the University of Northumbria, was built and the School became attached to the University of Durham. That University, lying close to the Cathedral, had been founded in 1834, largely for the religious education of Anglican clergy. The development of Newcastle as an important industrial city, briefly portrayed in Chapter 1, and the establishment in it of the 'Armstrong Building' (named after Sir William, later Lord A., the foremost entrepreneur in the area in the nineteenth century), meant that the scientific and engineering part of the University, to which the Medical School was attached, gradually overshadowed the section in Durham itself.

I myself, having had a public school education, good in itself but unsuitable for medicine, began my First M.B. studies in that Armstrong Building in 1930. They included Botany, Zoology and Organic Chemistry, but also the beginning of Anatomy and Physiology in the Medical School. We did not see a living patient for two years, but learned our anatomy very thoroughly. The rest of the course was centred on the Royal Victoria Infirmary (the R.V.I.). This structure, particularly well designed, had been opened by King Edward VII in 1904. I graduated in 1935 and, like most others, elected to attend the degree ceremony in Durham. My fellow graduates numbered 54 and included six Americans, all male, who had been unable to gain entry to a medical school in their own country. There were also six women and one male black African. In 1938 the Medical School moved into a new building closer to the R.V.I., irreverently called by its Dean, for architectural reasons, 'The Jam Factory'. Since then it has been superseded by another building actually attached to the R.V.I. The 'jam factory' now rather aptly houses Newcastle University's Department of Agriculture.

Meanwhile, after a most unseemly row over the sacking of a non-clini-cal Professor, which had overshadowed my student years and of which the late Mr E. M. Bettenson, former University Registrar, has given an excellent account, [1] a Royal Commission recommended that Durham University should be split into two divisions in the separate cities. This unsatisfactory state of affairs was subsequently changed into an arrange-ment for two entirely distinct Universities of Durham and Newcastle (not Northumbria), with great benefit to both.

In the faculty of medicine, before the introduction of the National Health Service (NHS) in 1948, the distinction between the Teaching and the Non-teaching hospitals was very significant. The former had great prestige, their consultant staff received no salary, but had to earn their living by private practice, and they had a monopoly of instructing the medical students. This last privilege doubtless subsequently helped their private practice. There was considerable competition to be elected to its staff. The R.V.I., the Fleming Memorial Hospital for Sick Children, and the Princess Mary Maternity were of this status in Newcastle. The non-teaching group comprised the Newcastle General Hospital (N.G.H.), Walkergate Fever Hospital, the Sanderson Orthopaedic Hos-pital, St Nicholas (mental) Hospital and an extraordinary structure in the middle of the Town Moor, kept ready and empty for decades waiting for cases of smallpox. They had been built and were maintained by the City Council through its Health Committee. The consultant staff were paid, had specified hours of duty and were permitted to engage in private practice. They did not, as a rule, teach medical students. However during the 12 years that he was Medical Officer of Health in the city, Dr John Charles and its Health Committee, through its chairman Alderman Sir Walter Thompson, steadily improved the status and quality of these hospitals. The consultant staff, still salaried, became of as good a standard as, if not better than, those in the R.V.I. and the patients they attracted for their private practice were just as discriminating. Only the buildings, especially some of those of the N.G.H., still recalled in appearance their 'Poor-law' origins. It was impossible to deny their suitability for the instruction of medical students, especially since the numbers of these were steadily rising.

When, therefore, after returning in 1945 from service in the Army overseas, I was in 1947 elected to the consultant staff of the R.V.I. as an assistant physician (but decided to specialise in heart disease), it was not difficult to form a satisfactory relationship with colleagues in the newly established Cardiovascular Department of the N.G.H. The principal obstacles were the physical distance of two miles and poor car parking facilities. If the account I have given in this volume appears unduly weighted in favour of my doings in the R.V.I., I hope that proper consideration will be given to those obstacles.

Finally, since in the first chapter of this account I have included a brief survey of Newcastle and its environs in the era when Sir William Hume, the founder of cardiology in the North-east, began practice, it seemed that an equally brief survey here of the contrast which today presents would not be inappropriate.

By 1992 Newcastle had become a very different city from what it was when this account of the heart disease in it began. Most of the changes are for the better, some for the reverse. Its traditional strengths, the export of coal (60% of whose energy still evaporates from the cooling towers of the country's power stations, to assist global warming), shipbuilding and heavy engineering have gone. Some promise of ship repairing has appeared in partial replacement, and Vickers make a precarious living building tanks for both the Ministry of Defence and export. But the most conspicuous and profitable replacements in the area have been the investments by Far Eastern (Japan, Korea and Taiwan) and German firms in motorcar construction and medium to light engineering. The standard of living has improved enormously, as has the health of the whole community. There is more social equality, and with the disappearance of the 'pit heaps', the countryside has again become so beautiful that a proportion of its inhabitants have begun to deprecate the success of the tourist industry. The North-east's castles, the most numerous in the country and genuine historic fortresses (relics of the constant warring between the Scots and English), are sometimes still occupied by the same families rather than managed by English Heritage or the National Trust. Instead of small colonies of Arabs and Chinese in South Shields and the City, there are now moderate-sized communities of Indians and Pakistanis settled on both sides of the nearly empty river. The downside is unemployment (better rather than worse as compared with the rest of Western Europe), resulting in more crime and vandalism, and a city skyline dominated by residential tower blocks in place of church towers and steeples. The University, released as we have seen from its former attachment to an ecclesiastical Durham, is now a large and comprehensive unit in its own right. The city's Polytechnic now has University status (of Northumbria).

Medically, as noted, the public's health is vastly improved, with heart disease at least as much better as everything else. Rheumatic valvular disease is less often encountered than it once was, but still more often than would be expected from the rarity of frank rheumatic fever. Coronary heart disease is at least as prevalent, probably because there are more old people about, cigarette smoking has only diminished a little, and neither a low calorie nor a non-atherogenic diet are popular. The finding that a small amount of alcohol each day can be beneficial has been welcomed with predictably untempered enthusiasm. Congenital malformations of the heart, for which once only sympathy could be offered, can now usually be totally corrected. The true prevalence of viral heart disease has not yet been truly assessed. To deal with all this, the city has three major hospitals, where perhaps it ought to have only two, and thirteen cardiologists, where in 1908 it had but one (Professor Hume). The facilities in the Cardiac Department of the Freeman Hospital are superb, and the use made of them first class.

Notes

1. Bettenson, E. M., The Hutchens Affair. *Durham University Journal,* 1982; 74: 159–98.

CHAPTER 1

THE ORIGIN AND DEVELOPMENT OF CARDIOLOGY IN NEWCASTLE

The first name that appears to link Newcastle with cardiology is that of Andrew Wilson MD, of Newcastle upon Tyne, who in 1774, when he was physician to the Infirmary, published *An Enquiry into the Moving Powers Employed in the Circulation of the Blood.* [1] But since, 100 years after Harvey's demonstration of the circulation of the blood, his conclusion was 'that the heart is not essentially and absolutely necessary to the circulation of body fluids,' the historian of Newcastle cardiology may register pleasure that he served for only three years (1772–1775) as Hon. Physician to the city's Infirmary before taking his speculative talents to London. Newcastle has much more reason to be proud of Byron Bramwell (1847–1931), who was born in Dockray Square, North Shields, qualified in Edinburgh, and after a period in general practice with his father in North Shields, became lecturer in medical jurisprudence at the Newcastle Orchard Street medical school in 1872. In 1874 he became physician and pathologist to the Infirmary. He left in 1879 (at the age of only 31) to become physician to the Royal Infirmary in Edinburgh. He was a brilliant teacher and returned to Newcastle on many occasions to lecture. Among his published works (very many of them neurological) is a textbook of 783 pages, entitled *Diseases of the Heart and Thoracic Aorta*. Much of the preparatory work on this must have been done in Newcastle, but it is scarcely reflected among his numerous contributions to *Proc Northumb Durh Med. Soc.* in the 1870s. A contemporary on the staff of the

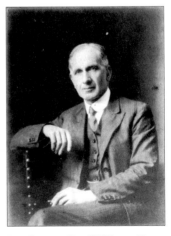

Professor Sir William Hume C.M.G., M.D. (Camb.), F.R.C.P., Hon. Physician, Royal Victoria Infirmary, Newcastle upon Tyne, 1908–44. Professor of Medicine, University of Durham.

Newcastle Infirmary, Sir David Drummond (1852–1932), was a general physician whom Hume greatly admired, and whose special interests were nervous and cardiovascular diseases. But it was with Professor Sir William Hume himself that cardiology in Newcastle effectively began. Son of George Haliburton Hume, surgeon on the staff of the Infirmary, he was educated in medicine at Cambridge and the London Hospital. He was appointed to the honorary staff of the Royal Victoria Infirmary in 1908 at 28 years of age, soon after the hospital had moved from its old position on Forth Banks behind Central Station high above the river, to its present site near the Town Moor, of which its land once formed part.

In 1908 Newcastle was at the peak of its prosperity. Ships from all over the world docked at its quayside, the swing-bridge opened daily to allow colliers up to load coal at Dunston Staithes and then to pass down again to carry it to London or to ports on the Continent. Where now Vickers' factory stands, Lord Armstrong's Elswick works were turning out every possible kind of armament for the British Army and for the British, Japanese and other navies of the world. Huge profits were made, of which the workers received a tiny share, and there was no unemployment. But by modern standards the health of the workforce was deplorable. Industrial injuries were common and uncompensated, tuberculosis and other infective ailments were rampant, and workers' children, if they did not succumb to the complications of measles and whooping cough, would not infrequently become deformed by rickets.

For anyone interested in heart disease, diphtheria and rheumatism in particular invited study. Diphtheria anti-toxin was available and used but there was no prevention and only too often children would present with a choking exudate on tonsils or larynx and a toxic myocarditis whose lethal consequences no amount of anti-toxin could avert. The one remarkable feature was that, if the victim did recover, he or she always did so completely and chronic diphtheritic myocarditis was not an entity. Rheumatism had three classical manifestations – acute rheumatism, commonly called rheumatic fever, with severe but transient arthritis, high fever with night sweats and erythematous rashes in the skin, or the neurological manifestations of chorea (St Vitus' Dance), which mercifully almost never coincided with polyarthritis, or, least obvious of all, 'growing pains' with slight or no fever, pains in muscles or joints with nothing to see and much debility. Any of the three was likely to be complicated or followed by valve disease. If the patient with acute rheumatism developed pericarditis, the accompanying pericardial effusion could be life-threatening, unless sucked out with a syringe.

Hume's interest in cardiology was evident at once and he made studies of cardiac dysrhythmias especially in diphtheria. He used the Mackenzie ink polygraph, which recorded simultaneously on clockwork-moved paper the pulsations of an artery at the wrist and of a vein in the neck. This at least was more convenient than the Marey polygraph with freshly smoked paper on a rotating drum which Sir James Mackenzie had initially used in his studies in general practice in Burnley many years before. Hume's publication in 1913 'A case in which a high speed of the auricles was not accompanied by a high speed of the

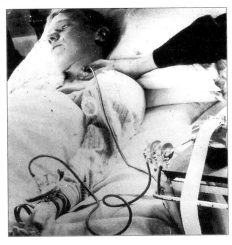

Dr W.E. Hume's Ink Polygraph. Adapted by Sir James Mackenzie (with help from Mr Shaw, watchmaker of Padiham) from Marey's Tambour and Dudgeon's Sphygmograph, to record simultaneously, on clockwork-driven paper, the pulsations of an artery at the wrist and a vein in the neck. The precursor of the Electrocardiograph.

ventricles' was one of the early descriptions of atrial flutter. In 1912 he persuaded the governing body of the hospital to purchase one of the new Einthoven galvanometers for taking electrocardiograms (E.C.Gs). It cost £250, a sum which hardly changed for the next 40 years.

The first electrocardiogram was of his house physician Charles H. Robson, taken on a falling photographic glass plate and, as can be seen in the illustration, was of excellent quality and normal. Sir John Charles, then a medical student, remembered the occasion, a 'Saturday morning and rather wet'. The next record was of a case of heart block. Hume wrote a small pamphlet about the instrument [2] and had soon established links with Sir Thomas Lewis at University College, London, Professor William Ritchie in Edinburgh and other pioneers. The First World War interrupted his studies, but through his friendship with Sir Bertrand Dawson (later Lord Dawson of Penn), whose house-physician he had been at the London Hospital, he was appointed Consulting Physician to the 1st Army and made records of the cardiac abnormalities in the cases of spirochaetal jaundice (a very dangerous rat-borne infection) which were occurring in some of the troops in the trenches.

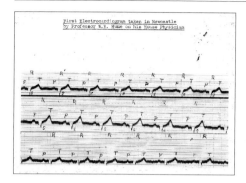

The first electrocardiogram, taken by Dr Hume on his house physician, Dr C.H. Robson, in 1912.

When the war was over he returned to the R.V.I. and developed cardiology further, but always within the framework of general medicine, of which all his working life he remained a superb practitioner. Two wards in the hospital, numbers 9 and 15, were linked up by electric wire and telephone, so that patients in their beds could have their E.C.Gs recorded, by now on celluloid, by the machine in the basement. It was an admirable system, but would have worked a little better if the excellent technician in the basement had not earned his nickname, 'Deafie' Thompson. Hume also acquired another instrument for his private practice and his secretary, Dillingham, his wife and other members of his own family became experts at developing and printing the records.

On the national front Hume had taken the lead in beginning the British Cardiac Society shortly after the war by writing in January 1922 to Cowan suggesting that he wrote to those other physicians in the country known to be interested in heart disease, proposing that they form a new organisation, the British Cardiac Club. The B.C.S. grew out of it, and Hume was a prominent and popular member of both, hosting meetings of the Society in Newcastle in 1926 and 1953. As his friend Sir John Parkinson once said, 'The room always seemed to light up a bit when Hume walked in'.

Locally of course his reputation also grew and he achieved a particularly high standing in the National Union of Mineworkers, whose cases for compensation he often supported in the courts. It cannot have been the privilege of many cardiologists in the UK to be able to go to the house of a miner who had just died and in whose case he was interested, perform a limited post-mortem in the bedroom, and be thanked by the widow as he left with the heart in his bag. He even had a technique for removing the heart via the rectum. As a teacher, not only of cardiology but, it seemed, of any branch of medicine, he was superb. He flouted the conventional rules of good lecturing by walking back and forth and peppering his discourse with innumerable 'ers', but the lucidity of that discourse, its common sense, its avoidance of technical jargon and the vivid illustrations from his own experiences made his lectures master-pieces. What student could forget the moment when he broke off his exposition and said 'I think it is time I told you one or two gruey stories'. He would then relate the case of the man lying in bed with a syphilitic aneurysm pulsating just beneath the skin of his upper chest, whilst his wife washed the floor with a cloth. Suddenly an arc of blood landed on the floor beside her. With enormous presence of mind, she clapped the floor-cloth on her husband's chest and staunched the flow. He was still just alive when Hume visited him the next day.

Hume took up the study of cardiology when treatment was neither very interesting nor very rewarding. Salicylates would do much for rheumatic symptoms but were not curative and would not prevent valvular disease. Digitalis had been introduced more than 100 years before by William Withering, who had himself worked out the principles of how it should be used, even if he did consider it had more effect on the kidneys than on the heart. Hume used the tincture, which had one merit over the tablets which superseded it, in that the dose could easily be modified to suit the patient. Of true diuretics, i.e. drugs which really worked on the kidneys, there were none until salyrgan and other organic compounds of mercury were introduced in 1919. Quinidine, the first drug after digitalis to modify the rhythm of the heart, became available in the same year. The interesting and rewarding challenges were in diagnosis and in under-standing the nature of disease. Sir James Mackenzie's adaptation of Marey's polygraph and his correlation of its recordings with long obser-vations of his patients' progress in general practice had revolutionised cardiology. The electrocardiograph was, however, a much more infor-mative tool and made it much easier to link the abnormalities seen *post mortem* in the heart with the rhythmic and the structural changes which had been seen in the E.C.G. Hume's museum classes, in which he correlated the patient's symptoms and signs and E.C.G. in life with the macro- and microscopic appearances at necropsy, were, in the opinion of Professor Nattrass and doubtless of generations of other students, the most brilliant of his achievements as a teacher.

Not surprisingly, those who had the privilege of being his house-physi-cians and registrars were proud of the experience, especially as he was always interested in and keen to facilitate their careers. Adrian Swan was one who learned a great deal of cardiology from him, and was much disappointed not to be elected to a vacancy on the staff of the R.V.I. which arose shortly before the Second World War. When Hume retired from

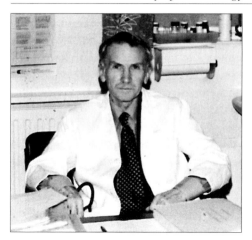

Dr Hewan A. Dewar M.D. (Durham), F.R.C.P. Consultant Cardiologist, Royal Victoria Infirmary and Freeman Hospital, Newcastle upon Tyne, 1947–78.

the honorary staff of that hospital in 1939 at the prescribed age of 60, there was no immediate successor to take charge of cardiology there until Hewan Dewar, with no previous special training in cardiology, inherited Hume's facilities and staff in the Royal Victoria Infirmary. It is difficult in these days of paid appointments in the NHS to realise how inevitably small these were. Between the wars Hume ran his male ward of 20 beds and his female of 10 with staff of one registrar and one house-physician. His assistant physician (latterly James Spence) by tradition was limited to four male and two female beds, for which the same junior staff served. The assistant physician's main commitment was to out-patients. Turn-over in the wards was not as rapid as today. A man with a major coronary thrombosis would spend a month in bed, the first week of it flat on his back, nourished through a feeding cup.

With a need to provide for his wife and five children entirely from private practice, and with a statutory obligation to the R.V.I. of only two mornings a week, it is astonishing how much Hume accomplished. But the physical legacy to the R.V.I. was one small room in the basement, with a screened off cubby-hole of a dark room, shared by two cardiographers and the hospital photographer. With the Cambridge string galvanometer, the E.C.G. was recorded on photo-sensitised celluloid from which, after development, a photographic print was made, mounted on paper and despatched without a report to the ward. A 3-lead E.C.G. took about 30 seconds to complete, a 12-lead one at least twice as long. Fortunately an early move to much more roomy though poorly ventilated premises, still in the basement, and the purchase of an American direct-writing E.C.G. machine enabled a much faster service to be provided, accompanied for the first time by a report.

In the meantime, however, Hume had been invited by Newcastle's Medical Officer of Health, Dr John Charles (later Chief Medical Officer

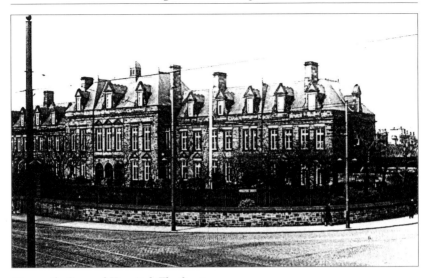

Newcastle General Hospital. The front.

to the Ministry of Health and knighted) to become physician, no longer honorary, at the Newcastle General Hospital, and remained on its staff from 1938 to 1949. There he was assisted by Paul Szekely,[3] a Czechoslovak refugee from Hitler, who had worked with the French cardiologist Laubry in Paris. Soon after the National Health Service was introduced in 1948, Hume, with his customary foresight, advised the Regional Health Authority to set up a Regional Cardiovascular Unit at the New-castle General Hospital. Adrian Swan, who had returned from the war and already had a post at the N.G.H., was the obvious choice as head of it. It began functioning in 1951. Working with Swan were his deputy, Frederic Jackson,[4] a London Hospital graduate who developed a special interest in ischaemic heart disease, Paul Szekely whose many research papers, especially on rheumatic heart disease and heart disease in pregnancy, are recorded elsewhere in this account, and Charles Henderson, a Durham graduate, who had recently returned from the U.S.A., where with a Nuffield Fellowship he had been studying various aspects of cardiology, including in particular ballistocardiography. This was a technique for assessing the mechanical function of the heart by recording the successive tailward and headward movement of the whole body as the blood was pumped, first to the arch of the aorta and then to the legs. Like apex cardiography, which attracted his interest a few years later, it never gave as much reliable information as its ingenuity had led people to expect and its vogue was short. Equally disappointing was the

N.G.H.'s first strain-gauge manometer for cardiac catheter work, which Henderson nursed most carefully during his air journey back from the USA. The manufacturers had supplied it already ruined by a puncture.

Nevertheless Henderson became a deft manipulator of that very valuable tool, the cardiac catheter, both at the N.G.H. and also in the surgical unit at Shotley Bridge. He and Jackson performed most of the investigative procedures which had to precede operation on the numerous cases of rheumatic, valvular and congenital heart disease which the Cardiovascular Unit attracted from all over the Northern Region. Marion Bethune's contribution in paediatric cardiology is described later.

These developments took place because in 1928 or 1929 there had occurred in Germany an event whose enormous importance to cardiology lay largely unrecognised for 14 or 15 years. Wilhelm Forssmann, a very junior doctor working in the 2nd medical department of the Krankenhaus Moabit in Berlin, engaged in a personal experiment. Realising that anything introduced into a vein in the arm must end up in the right atrium of the heart, he thought that it would be interesting to see if a ureteric catheter (a fine tube usually passed via the bladder up towards

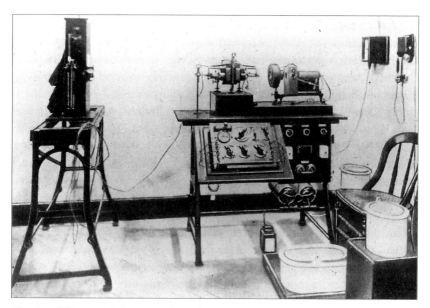

The Royal Victoria Infirmary's first electrocardiograph instrument, used between 1912 and 1948. The current from 3 different aspects of the beating heart were led in turn from 2 of the baths of saline, into which both arms and one leg had been placed, through a quartz fibre (the "string"), suspended between two powerful magnets. A strong light threw silhouettes of deflections of the fibre on to a falling photographic glass plate, which was then developed.

a kidney) would do just that. So he lubricated one with olive oil and, under a local anaesthetic, inserted it into a vein at his elbow and pushed it on. He then walked to the X-ray department and confirmed that it was indeed in the right atrium. He suffered no ill-effects and demonstrated the procedure to a more senior assistant, who then reported it to his chief. The latter offered no opinion but suggested that he should discuss the matter with the University Professor (G. Klemperer), head of the 1st Medical Department. The great man found the experiment interesting, of some value perhaps for research, but not of clinical interest. There the matter was left, no encouragement was given, and Forssmann went off to the USA, presumably to study urology, in which he subsequently had a career in his own country. He did however publish his experiment in 1929 under the title 'Die sonderung des rechten Herzenszone' in *Klin Wchnschr. 8,2085* [Personal communication to H.A.D. from Dr F. L. Kronenberger of Sunderland, who was a friend of the assistant]. There was some follow-up by various workers, but it was probably André Cournand,[5] who in New York in 1941 did most to introduce the technique into clinical practice. In the UK McMichael and Sharpey-Schafer soon followed suit, and with the war over, clinicians were able to exploit it further. By measuring pressures and taking samples of blood for estimation of oxygen content from (ultimately) all chambers of the heart and (later) injecting radio-opaque fluids through it, they and others were able to obtain just the information which surgeons needed before they could proceed to curative and palliative treatments.

Soon, therefore, after he was appointed to the consultant staff of his hospital, Dewar paid a visit to London to learn from Frances Gardner at the Royal Free Hospital how it was done. He met her at the Royal Free but had to travel with her to another hospital, clutching in the front passenger seat the 'manometer', a long glass tube which projected through the sunshine roof. Back in Newcastle he substituted an aneroid manometer from a B.P. machine and in 1949, assisted by T. A. Grimson, he performed the first cardiac catheterisation in the North. Soon, with the help of Charles Warrick and later of Peter Hacking, the R.V.I. radiologists, he was able to provide a full investigative service of cardiac catheterisation and angiocardiography.

These investigative procedures had, as we have seen, assumed particular importance because of the development of cardiac surgery, of which an account is given separately. Because they were necessary before operation in a large proportion of cases, though not all, and the apparatus was expensive, most of the cases in the Northern Region had to be seen by a cardiologist and admitted to the R.V.I. the N.G.H. or Shotley Bridge. Accordingly, the cardiologists began paying visits, mostly every one or two months, to the various general hospitals in the region to see new cases and follow-ups. These visits were at the invitation of the physicians in these hospitals with whom, as Hume had foreseen, they had formed friendships in the Newcastle Cardiac Club and the Association of Physicians of Region No. 1 – both organisations which Hume had founded. The Regional Health Authority defrayed the travelling expenses.

It is interesting that another and equally valuable technique for diagnosis began to be introduced into cardiology about 10 years later, but took a curiously long time to become universally adopted. Echocardiography is the term used to describe the transmission of high-frequency sound waves, which penetrate and bounce back from the various structures of the heart and great vessels, to be picked up by a receiver and converted into images on a fluorescent screen. Derived from sonar (Asdic), a method of detecting submarines in warfare, ultrasound has long been widely used in industry and various branches of medicine, especially obstetrics. The difficulty with the heart is that much of it is surrounded by the air-containing lungs, which of course convey sounds no better than do double-glazed windows. But part of the heart is close to the chest wall and it can be 'accessed' from other aspects above and below (and even behind) as will be described in the chapter on paediatric research. The Japanese became interested in its use for heart disease in the early 1950s and the Swedes and Germans soon followed, with the U.S.A. not far behind, in the 1960s. The British, the most menaced by submarines in the Second World War, were not in the forefront of the development of echocardiography! They have, however, caught up since.

Examination of the patient by echocardiography is painless, safe, much quicker than catheter studies, and easily repeatable. Interpreting the shadows, however, requires some study, skill and experience. Dewar obtained an echo instrument for his department in the early 1970s but, nearing retirement himself, never became confident in its use. His Senior Registrar, Gordon Terry, later appointed a Consultant in Durham, however, soon became very proficient and Dewar's successor at the R.V.I., Roger Hall, arrived even more so. The cardiologists at the Freeman Hospital, especially the paediatricians, took it up about the same time. The instrument, not too expensive, is also very suitable for those general physicians in Regional Hospitals who have a special interest in heart disease. The information obtained by echocardiography often makes cardiac catheter studies unnecessary, and is particularly valuable for follow-up examinations.

Meanwhile, the units at the R.V.I. and the N.G.H. were to some extent in friendly rivalry, each keen to keep abreast of new developments. They were not in local competition for money, because funding of the cardiology unit at the R.V.I. came from its Board of Governors, which was financed directly from the Department of Health in London, but which also had use of the hospital's endowment fund, dating from its days as a voluntary hospital. The Regional Cardiovascular Unit at the N.G.H. was financed by the Regional Health Authority, whose funds, also provided by the Department of Health, had to service the whole Region. A weekly review of the cases investigated, held in the Department of Radiology in the N.G.H., provided an excellent opportunity for mutual discussion and shared experience. It was particularly valuable in relation to congenital heart disease for Dr Marion Bethune (later Farmer), the first paediatric cardiologist, worked closely with both units. There was also some collaboration in research. Swan and Dewar did write a joint paper in 1952 on 'The Heart in Haemochromatosis'[6] but the latter's enthusiasm for fibrinolysis, which began in 1961 with the 'Fibrinolytic Treatment of Coronary Thrombosis – a pilot study',[7] was not echoed in the C.V.S. unit. Dewar, however, was honorary secretary of the Association of Physicians of Region No. 1 for 27 years following its inception in 1950, and thus was able to recruit physicians from throughout the Region in a collaborative (and negative) project on steroid therapy in acute myocardial infarction[8] and in a trial of clofibrate (a cholesterol-reducing drug) in the treatment of ischaemic heart disease which began in 1968[9] and finished simultaneously with a similar Scottish trial in 1971.

The late 1960s and the 1970s were a time of very important changes in the treatment of heart disease. Julian, while in Edinburgh, had put forward in an article in the *Lancet* the idea that patients who had a heart attack would be better cared for in a 'coronary care unit', i.e. in a group of beds with special facilities. A fuller description of such units and how they evolved in Newcastle is given in Chapter 2. That chapter also deals with the problem of how patients can be conveyed to such units with the least possible delay, a problem which intensified a few years later when a method of dissolving the clots in their coronary arteries was devised. These were exciting times.

The same period also saw substantial improvement in heart surgery for both congenital and acquired heart abnormalities and these are more amply set forth in Chapter 6, where the temporary split into two units,

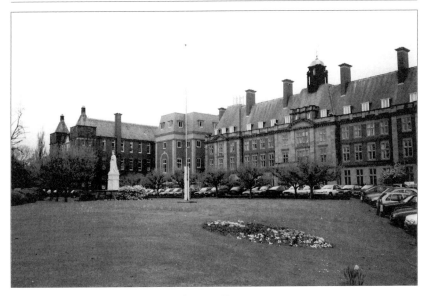

Royal Victoria Infirmary, Newcastle upon Tyne.

both about 15 miles from Newcastle, is described. In 1974, when the British Cardiac Society again had its annual meeting in Newcastle, this time under the joint chairmanship of Hewan Dewar and Fred Jackson, representing the two main cardiac medical centres, surgery was still split. But help was in sight. After years of discussion, the decision was finally taken to build an entirely new hospital, the 'Freeman'. [10] The Newcastle General, which had started as a poor-law institution, had been built, for reasons perhaps best not investigated, in front of a large cemetery and there was no other possible building site in the area. The Royal Victoria Infirmary might have been given further land by the Corporation and the Freemen of the City, as had been done at the time of the Queen's Jubilee in 1897, but underneath the grass of the possible site lay old coal-mine workings as well as a little-known tunnel through which the coal used once to be conveyed to the river's quays. So the new hospital was a sound concept and for cardiology a wonderful development. At last both medical and surgical aspects of it would be concentrated in the same area. It was a pity that the new children's hospital was going to have to be built adjoining the R.V.I.

Strangely, the new Freeman Hospital was conceived by the Regional planners as a District General Hospital serving the eastern end of the city. Since it had no Accident and Emergency department, and the decision had already been taken to position within it a cardiovascular unit serving the whole Region, the concept was not realistic. After much discussion, at times rather heated, the hospital was recognised as an integral part of Newcastle's Teaching Group. The worst error, which could be only partly corrected, was the total omission of a Coronary Care Unit. It transpired that an eminent general physician member of the Project Team had advised the Health Authority that none was needed as the patients could be cared for perfectly adequately on the general wards! A hurried revision of the plans resulted in the present site of the C.C.U. about a quarter of a mile and two floors distant from the Cardiac Theatres and Catheter Laboratories.

With the expansion of cardiac surgery and the need for specialist assessment, to be followed later by complicated in-patient investigations prior to operation, the cardiological clinics already established in most of the Regional hospitals, and now sometimes also attended by surgeons, proved particularly valuable. They saved the patients and the ambulance services a very great deal of unnecessary travel.

The year 1975 saw what was probably the most momentous event for cardiology in Newcastle, the appointment of a full-time Professor. It came about because the University had, in the early 1970s, approached the British Heart Foundation, a charitable body, with a proposal to create a Chair of Cardiology which would be based at the Freeman Hospital, then under construction. The Heart Foundation agreed to fund the salary of a Professor and a Lecturer, together with modest running expenses, on the understanding that the University would provide accommodation and support services in the new hospital. Through a generous anonymous donation, it was possible to construct an addition to the original designs for the Cardiothoracic Centre, by filling in an open space that had been planned under the Intensive Care Unit. This provided enough space for offices for the Professor and his staff, as well as two laboratory areas.

Professor Desmond Julian, who for the last 10 years had been Consultant Physician in the Royal Infirmary, Edinburgh, was appointed Professor of Cardiology and took up his appointment in January 1975 at the age of 48. A graduate of Cambridge and the Middlesex Hospital, London, he had trained in cardiology at the National Heart Hospital, London (under Dr Paul Wood), the Peter Bent Brigham Hospital, Boston, and Edinburgh. In 1961 he was the first to put forward the concept of the coronary care unit (the siting of a small number of beds with special equipment and specially trained medical and nursing staff) in an article in the *Lancet*. [11] In 1961, he went to Sydney, Australia, to set up a coronary care unit virtually simultaneously with those in Kansas, Philadelphia, and Toronto,

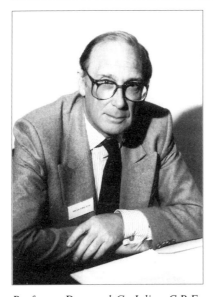

Professor Desmond G. Julian C.B.E., B.A., M.D. (Cantab. and Gothenburg), F.R.C.P. (Ed., Lond and Australia), British Heart Foundation Professor of Cardiology, University of Newcastle, 1975–86. Ex-President of the Brit. Card. Soc.

and returned to Edinburgh in 1964 as Consultant Physician at the Royal Infirmary. He was already a Fellow of the Edinburgh, London and Australian Colleges of Physicians, the author of a large number of original papers and writer or editor of many textbooks, including several editions of his own *Cardiology*. His arrival in Newcastle, therefore, brought the Medical School considerable prestige. When Fred Jackson retired in 1977, he bought Fred's house in Darras Hall and was not a little surprised to find that the purchase included a donkey which Fred had bought as an unexpected (and unappreciated) birthday present for his own wife! But Fred, a keen traveller and mountaineer, had always been resourceful.

Widowed with two teenage children, Desmond was fortunate in having already on the nursing staff of the Newcastle General Hospital his own married sister, able to help him on social occasions, even if one of these, a musical evening, was so audibly successful that the neighbours invited the police also to attend! His own combination of intellect, charm and kindness with firmness made him a most successful head of the new professional department.

Initially, he worked in the Cardiology Department in Newcastle General Hospital, and continued to do so until Freeman Hospital was fully open in 1977. The opening in that year was celebrated by an International Conference on Arrhythmias which was attended by many of the world leaders in that field.

In the Cardiac Department of the N.G.H. he found that there already existed close cooperation between cardiologists, cardiac surgeons and anaesthetists and the Regional Physics Department, headed by Professor Frank Farmer. This was not only about the design of new, and adaptation of existing, equipment such as cardiac monitors, but there had also been research projects. One of the most valuable of these had been the development by Andrew Pay of a computer system for the 'real-time' measurement and recording of pressures inside the heart during its catheterisation. This was used with varying degrees of enthusiasm and understanding by the cardiologists and sadly fell into disuse with the demise of the computer hardware for which the programmes had been written.

At the Freeman Hospital Professor Julian was joined by Dr R. W. F. Campbell, who had also come from Edinburgh by way of the Department of Cardiology of Duke University, North Carolina, where he had gained expertise in arrhythmology, and by the medical physicist, Dr Alan Murray. Together their research work concentrated on myocardial infarction and arrhythmias. Computerised methods of arrhythmia detection were developed, which permitted detailed examination of the arrhythmias which complicate myocardial infarction, and of the effectiveness of anti-arrhythmic drugs. With the support of Professor Boddy (Farmer's successor in Medical Physics), a branch of that department was established in the Freeman Hospital with Alan Murray as its head. He and his colleagues in that department and the University Department of Computer Engineering developed the Hospital's ambulatory E.C.G. service, the cable link between the C.C.U. and the Professorial Cardiac Unit, the radio link between that Unit and the paramedics, and the establishment of another diagnostic tool, the Thallium Stress Test. Altogether a most useful combination of service and research, well described in a number of publications.

The Cardiovascular Department also acted as the base for a large secondary trial of sotalol (a beta blocker) after myocardial infarction which has been a landmark study in this field.[12] The Department was also early in the field of thrombolytic drugs, participating in the trials of streptokinase, anistreplase and tissue plasminogen activator.

The University and NHS Departments of Cardiology worked closely with each other, with Dr Fred Jackson, Dr Charles Henderson and later Dr Ron Gold successively holding the position of administrative head of the NHS Department. Members of the University Department played their role in the routine cardiological services of the hospital, whilst NHS staff participated in teaching and research. As a consequence, new advances in cardiology were rapidly adopted. Thus Professor Julian had met Andreas Grüntzig shortly after he had published his original paper on coronary angioplasty[13] (a method of widening a coronary artery by inflating a very small balloon introduced through a catheter), and shortly thereafter Dr Douglas Reid and Dr David Williams attended one of Grüntzig's master classes on the technique in Zurich.

Meanwhile, significant retirements had taken place. Selwyn Griffin's unit at Seaham Hall closed, when Freeman Hospital opened in 1977, and he himself retired the next year on his 65th birthday, Hedley Brown taking his place. In 1977, some two and a half years before his 65th birthday, Fred Jackson left the Newcastle General Hospital for Patterdale in Cumbria. There, his resourcefulness unimpaired, he decided to help the Mountain Rescue Team in their work. His most remarkable contribution to that remarkable organisation's exploits was to apply both mouth-to-mouth respiration and external cardiac compression to a collapsed man all the way from the site of his collapse to the Cumberland Infirmary in Carlisle. There the heartbeat was successfully restarted, though sadly the recovery of the brain was not so satisfactory. At the N.G.H. his post was taken by Keith Evemy. In 1978 Dewar retired at 65 from his appointment at the Royal Victoria Infirmary but continued some animal and laboratory research and also took over from Dr Tony Spriggs the running of Northern ASH, the anti-smoking organisation. His successor was Dr R. J. C. Hall, a very well-trained cardiologist from London. Responding to both the need for economy and the opportunity of superb apparatus there, Roger performed his 'special procedures', viz. cardiac catheters, angiograms and insertion of pacemakers at the newly opened Freeman Hospital, but otherwise continued to work at the R.V.I., where he had some useful extensions made to the department. However, nine years later he decided to move to another consultant appointment in Cardiff. Philip Adams was his successor.

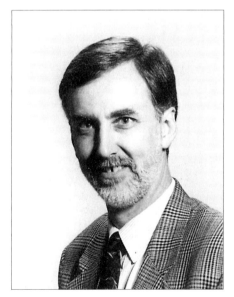

Dr Philip C. Adams, B.A. (Oxon), M.B., B.S. (Newc.), F.R.C.P., Consultant Cardiologist, Royal Victoria Infirmary and Freeman Hospital, Newcastle, 1987–.

Professor Julian, who had been elected President of the British Cardiac Society in 1985, retired from the Chair the following year to take up the position of Medical Director of the British Heart Foundation.

Julian was succeeded in 1986 by Professor Ronald W. F. Campbell, aged 40, who had been Julian's first assistant. An Edinburgh graduate, he had been trained in cardiology both there and in the U.S.A. He was already carrying out research into disturbances of the rhythm of the heart and continued it after Julian's departure. It formed the main thrust of work in the department. A fuller account will be given in the chapter headed 'Research'. Research, indeed, remains the main part of his work, as befits a University Professor, especially one financed by the British Heart Foundation, but his influence is easily seen in most other chapters of this story.

The policy, already mentioned, whereby members of the University Department play a part in the routine cardiological services of the hospital whilst the NHS staff participate in teaching and research, has continued. With time the actual persons involved have naturally changed. Of the NHS staff, David Williams came in 1975 from Birmingham with an appropriate interest in arrhythmias and Douglas Reid has shown a similar one in fibrinolytic treatment of coronary thrombosis. They form, with the addition in 1987 of Rodney Bexton, the backbone of those 'routine cardiological services'. The senior lecturers in the University have been Philip Adams,[14] Janet McComb, John Bourke, and Steve Furniss. The first two now hold NHS consultant appointments, but their commitment to research is undiminished. The publications of all four have contributed substantially to the categories of research summarised in the Research Chapter of this work. The copies of the annual Staff Returns to the B.H.F., reproduced with Professor Campbell's permission in the Appendices, also give the names of the many

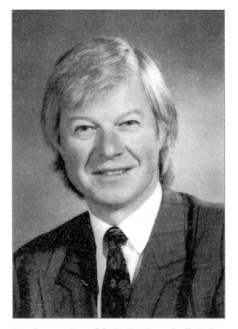

Professor Ronald W.F. Campbell B.Sc., M.B., Ch.B. (Ed), F.R.C.P. (Ed., Lond., and Glas.) British Heart Foundation Professor of Cardiology, Newcastle, 1986–. Pres. Brit. Card. Soc., 1997.

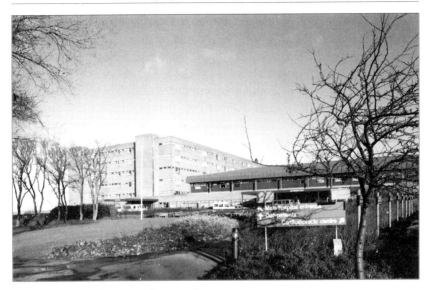

Freeman Hospital, Newcastle upon Tyne.

others who have in the department contributed to those categories and then moved elsewhere. Quite a proportion still remain in contact.

The finances of the department are interesting. We have already noted that it was the University of Newcastle which approached the British Heart Foundation for funds to establish the Chair of Cardiology, presumably because it was not given enough money by the government to set it up on its own. The University's contribution is to pay the rates and a service charge and it also makes a modest and variable annual grant, which ranges between one and a few tens of thousands of pounds. The NHS, through its grant to the Freeman Hospital, a Trust Hospital, pays the salary of one secretary and generously allows some of the consultant cardiologists both in the Teaching Group and in the Region to spend a little time which they can spare from routine duties to participate in research. It has also permitted the Medical Physics Department of the Teaching Group to play an absolutely essential part in this research. Unfortunately the recent reforms of the NHS, calculated to save money, have tended to hinder rather than to help that research. Thus, although the Cardiology Department has benefited from much good will and modest help from this combination of University, British Council and NHS, far and away the largest contribution to finance has come from the British Heart Foundation. Most of the research is actually carried out by research assistants, each of whom has to apply annually for its renewal, for few are completed in one year. Other research assistants from overseas have been funded by the British Council or by their own governments, or have paid for themselves. A number of medical students have also taken part in research as a feature of their studies for a degree in Medical Science. A relatively modest proportion of the money has been sought from the pharmaceutical industry. The objective of some of the research has been to enable patients to live without drugs! Never in the history of cardiology in Newcastle has so much research of the highest quality been carried out, and the public, who benefit from it, may also congratulate themselves that it is not from taxation but by their own forward-looking support for the British Heart Foundation that funds are available. As one vigorous research worker said to one of the authors, 'If I ever get into desperate straits for money, I appeal to the public and they respond'.

Notes

1. In Wilson's *Medical researches: being a enquiry into the nature and origin of hysterics in the female constitution, and into the distinction between that disease and hypochondriac or nervous disorders . . .* 1776 (copies BL and Wellcome) there is the 'Substance of a lecture delivered at Newcastle, 28th December, 1773, on the natural powers employed in the circulation of the blood, independent of the action of the heart'. In this Wilson proposes the reactionary theory: ' . . . not to disprove that it is by the action of the heart that the blood is thrown out into the arteries . . . but . . . that these actions have little or no concern in supporting the progress of the blood along the finer arteries . . . still less . . . on its motion through the veins back again to the heart'. He quotes Whytt on 'perceptual oscillations of the finer vessels, squeezing the blood forward in the direction of its progress . . . ' and concludes that the heart is not 'essentially and absolutely necessary to the circulation of our fluids'. Gardner-Medwin.
2. Hume W. E., Demonstration of the electrocardiograph. *Univ. Durh. Coll. Med. Gaz.* 1913–4; 14:75.
3. Appointed house physician 1941, registrar 1942, consultant 1948.
4. Appointed 1950, retired 1977.
5. Cournand A., Ranges H. A., Recording of right heart pressures in man. *Proc. Soc. Exp. Biol. & Med.* 1941; 46: 34–6.
6. Swan W. G. A., Dewar H. A., The heart in haemochromatosis. *Brit. Heart J.* 1952; 14: 117–24.
7. Dewar H. A., Horler A. R., Cassells-Smith A. J., Fibrinolytic treatment of coronary thrombosis: a pilot study. *BMJ* 1961; 2: 671–5.
8. A group of physicians in the Newcastle Region. Steroid therapy in acute myocardial infarction: A controlled trial. *Newc. Med. J.* 1968; 30: 82–9.

9. Group of Physicians of Newcastle upon Tyne Region (Organising secretary Dewar H. A.) Trial of Clofibrate in the treatment of ischaemic heart disease. *BMJ* 1971; 4: 767–75.

10. The word Freeman, which crops up from time to time, derives from the days when various crafts and trades in the city had their own representatives with certain rights, separate from those of the Mayor and Corporation. The most important of these is that the latter own the Town Moor, but not its herbage. The Freemen own the grass and each of them has the right to graze two milch cows on it. The possibility of disagreement between the two bodies has greatly helped to preserve the integrity of the Moor itself.

11. Julian D. G., Treatment of cardiac arrest in acute myocardial ischaemia and infarction. *Lancet* 1961; 2: 840–4.

12. Reduction of mortality after myocardial infarction with long-term beta-adrenergic blockade. A Multinational International study. *Brit. Med. J.* 1977; 2: 419–21.

13. Gruntzig A. Transluminal dilatation of coronary stenosis. *Lancet* 1978; 1: 263 [letter].

14. P. C. Adams is a graduate of Oxford and Newcastle, and has studied cardiology in both the UK and the U.S.A. He took up his appointment as cardiologist at the R.V.I. in 1987 and has facilities and duties at the Freeman Hospital. There he performs the technical investigations of his own patients and also shares with Rodney Bexton the duties of inserting the pacemakers for the area. But his main duties are in the R.V.I. There he is responsible for an extremely busy coronary care unit, where technical advances are so frequent that his bulletin of instructions for staff is now number 22! He also trains paramedics and teaches medical students, has set up a rehabilitation unit for the patients, and is very active in research – so active, in fact, that in 15 years he has written 43 papers as well as reviews and chapters in books. The research has included trials of thrombolytic and other drugs and, perhaps most importantly of all his current investigations, into the factors responsible for the development of coronary atherosclerosis.

The financial support for his research comes from the B.H.F. and local private funds.

CHAPTER 2

PREVENTION AND
MANAGEMENT OF HEART ATTACKS

There are a number of heart and blood vessel conditions from which a patient may suddenly die. Deformities of the aortic valve, some diseases of the heart muscle (myocarditis, cardiomyopathy), rupture or dissection of the aorta are examples, but disease (atherosclerosis) of the heart's own arteries, the coronaries, is much the most frequent and the best known. That the precipitating factor for sudden death may be a surge of adrenalin into the bloodstream is also no surprise to animal physiologists. Nor is the fact that the secretion of the adrenalin is often the consequence of emotion. The great surgeon and anatomist, John Hunter in the 18th century, who had angina, declared, 'My life is in the hands of any rascal who puts me in a rage'. The accuracy of his statement was numerically confirmed in Newcastle in 1975.[1] Dr Allan Myers, now Consultant Physician in Blackburn but then Senior House Officer at the Royal Victoria Infirmary in Newcastle, questioned the close relatives and observers of 100 patients in the Newcastle area, who had died suddenly of their coronary disease, about the exact circumstances in which the disaster had occurred. The most significant of several was indeed acute psychological stress. It is worth noting that the 'stress' was quite often pleasurable, and it is perhaps a sign of the times in which we live that in two cases the pleasure came from notification that the decree for a long-awaited divorce had just been made absolute. Similarly, a favourite story of Hume's, many years before, was of three patients, whom he saw in one afternoon, all suffering from angina. He made it his practice never to offer prognoses, but as he dictated the letters to his secretary, he remarked that if he had had to offer them he would have given the best to the last patient, who was on the point of retirement to a life of rest and indulgence in his hobbies. In fact the man had died on his way home from the consultation. Myers might have concluded that it was the intensity of delight at his prospects that was his undoing.

In Hume's day there was no effective means of either prevention or of treatment. The almost universal practice, to which attention has already been drawn, of putting a patient with a major coronary thrombosis to bed for a month, the first week of it with him lying on his back, was presumably an attempt to reduce the work of the heart and so limit the risk of its failure and sudden death. If the patient did, nevertheless, suddenly die, efforts at resuscitation almost always failed.

As is so often the case in medicine, it was only when certain assumptions and practices, apparently so logical, were challenged, that progress was made. Firstly estimates of cardiac output made with the help of the cardiac catheter showed that when somebody lies flat on his back his heart has more, not less, work to do. The next challenges were to certain well established practices and most of them were made in the remarkable decade 1960 to 1970. Some years before that it had been shown that mouth-to-mouth (or mouth-to-nose) respiration was a far more effective way of delivering air into the lungs than the old methods of Schafer and Sylvester, so painstakingly taught to generations of first-aid workers. It is also very much less tiring. But however great the improvement, for true efficiency this artificial respiration must be followed as soon as possible by 'intubation', i.e. the insertion of a tube into the windpipe, a procedure used by anaesthetists since the 1930s. Through it pure oxygen can be blown if required. Then in 1960 Kouwenhoven and colleagues in Baltimore[3] published a new way of making the non-contracting heart eject blood by compressing it between breastbone and spine. It was they who labelled this forceful procedure 'massage'. The amount ejected is about a fifth of the normal. The immediate forerunner of the method, 'open-heart massage', in which the chest was opened surgically and the heart squeezed manually, had rarely been accomplished with success.

The improved circulation into the coronary and other arteries induced by this 'closed-chest massage' is also sometimes enough to enable the heart to start beating again on its own. When it does not do so, then an electrical shock may do the trick. It had long been known from animal experiments, and more recently from continuous ECG recordings in man, that most often the heart had not stopped altogether (asystole), but was fibrillating, i.e. twitching irregularly, rapidly and ineffectually. An electric shock would terminate this. Here again there was room for improvement. The kind of shock previously used had been with an alternating current, and this was apt to be followed by some damage to the muscle of the heart. In 1963,[4] however, Lown and colleagues in Boston, U.S.A. showed that a direct current shock, given from a rechargeable capacitor, caused far less damage. Now when required, such a device is used routinely. If asystole does occur, then a single thump on the chest or cardiac compression may restart it, but an electric shock is more likely to do so. Given through the exposed tip of an insulated wire inserted like a cardiac catheter via a vein into the inside of the heart, the stimuli are more effective, require a lower voltage, and are virtually painless.

Meanwhile in 1961 Desmond Julian, later Professor of Cardiology in Newcastle but then Senior Registrar in Edinburgh, suggested the setting up of 'coronary care units', that is to say the designating in each hospital of a group of beds, supplied with special equipment and specially trained medical and nursing staff.[5] The same year he was invited to set one up in Australia and a few others were started in North America about the same time. The concept was presently adopted, perhaps rather slowly, world-wide.

In Newcastle the first C.C.U. was started in the Royal Victoria Infirmary in 1968 with four beds in a general ward soon replaced by four sidewards converted and specially equipped for the purpose. Since the number of daily admissions was more than the adjacent general ward could subsequently handle, and the greatest risk had passed after 48 hours, most of the cases admitted to the C.C.U. were after that period transferred to the care of the physician who was on receiving duty on the day of their admission. An emergency system for the whole hospital was also introduced, whereby, on receipt of a telephone call with a priority number, a nurse and doctor from the C.C.U. and an anaesthetist ran with emergency equipment to the site of the collapse. The service proved efficient in respect of the speed with which the team reached the patient, but the number of permanently successful resuscitations was disappointingly small. At the Newcastle General Hospital, through the generosity of Mr Lionel Jacobson, a specially built C.C.U. unit of 10 beds was opened in 1969.

Both units were modified as improvements in treatments

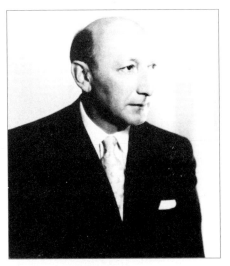

Lionel Jacobson Esq. M.A., D.C.L., Benefactor to Cardiac Departments of Royal Victory Infirmary and Newcastle General Hospital.

were introduced. That in the R.V.I. now functions in new premises and has its own post-C.C.U. ward. It takes a large proportion of the cases of coronary thrombosis which occur in and near the city. When the Regional Cardiology Department moved to Freeman Hospital in 1978, the C.C.U. at N.G.H. ceased to function as a true C.C.U. but after the appointment of Dr Keith Evemy there in 1983, the unit resumed its original role, but on a reduced scale with only four beds. It is due to close in 1997 when the function of the N.G.H. substantially alters.

With the opening of the ten-bedded C.C.U. at Freeman Hospital, with its adjacent 27-bed Post-Coronary Care ward, a new concept of patient care was introduced. The cardiologists are on a roster to be on call for, and in charge of, the unit for a week at a time. New patients admitted during that week remain under the care of that consultant for the whole of their admission period and also for their subsequent follow-up. The C.C.U. has 10 acute beds and 27 more in the adjacent Post-C.C.U. part. The nursing staff, from their centrally placed station, can see the monitoring screens of 16 patients. The 27 patients in the remainder of the ward include not only patients who have been transferred from the acute section, but also less urgent cases ('unstable angina'), patients who need pacemakers or who have just had one installed, patients just discharged from the surgical Intensive Care Unit after their heart operation, and

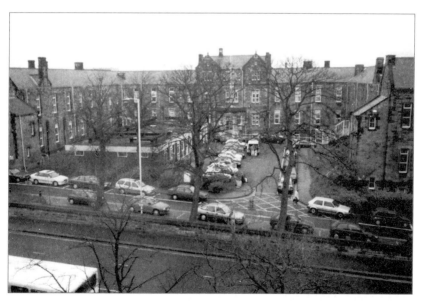

Newcastle General Hospital. The Coronary Care Unit (single-storey) is in the middle.

others being investigated for their need and fitness for such surgical treatment. The staff also provide for emergencies occurring elsewhere in the hospital. The R.V.I. and the Freeman both provide a rehabilitation service managed by nurses and dietitians, and both take part in the 'on the spot' teaching of medical students.

Meanwhile, in 1964, another most important advance in prevention and treatment took place in the discovery of the 'beta-blocking drugs'. The first satisfactory one of these was devised by Sir James Black of Imperial Chemical Industries in 1964, and its beneficial effect on angina was described by Srivastava *et. al.* in the R.V.I. in the same year. [6] But the anti-arrhythmic properties were every bit as valuable. Black's knighthood and Nobel Prize were well deserved. The beta-blockers have saved many, many lives. But all drugs of real value have so-called side effects and this group is no exception. That first one is still in use, and several Newcastle physicians from both main hospitals took a part in the clinical trials which established its remarkable properties. [7]

Its successor, Practolol, had even better properties and the cardiologists in Newcastle, and in a great many other centres in the world, were happy to contribute patients to a controlled trial. This showed that the drug substantially reduced mortality if it were taken for the next year after a heart attack. Only when the trial was completed did it become apparent that a very small percentage of those who took the drug would develop damage to their eyes and other organs. It was promptly abandoned. The value of another beta-blocker, sotalol, manufactured by a different firm, free from this 'side-effect', and used for the same purpose, was established by Julian, Jackson, Szekely and Prescott in 1983. [8]

The properties of other drugs for preventing rhythm disturbances of the heart have also been tested in Newcastle and elsewhere. The remarkable ability of aspirin to prevent thrombosis and rethrombosis in diseased coronary arteries has been confirmed and put into regular practice.

Meanwhile another development still had taken place in Belfast. An obstetrical Flying Squad, devised by Professor Farquhar Murray, had been operating in Newcastle for 30 years, and in 1965 Dewar, in an article in *The Practitioner*, [9] had suggested that something similar might be introduced for cases of coronary thrombosis. But it was J. F. Pantridge, Consultant Cardiologist in the Royal Victoria Hospital, Belfast, who first set up a coronary ambulance. This is a remarkable and efficient way of delivering emergency methods of observation and treatment to patients in the place where they are first needed, i.e. the home, the workplace or wherever the patient has taken ill. He started his coronary ambulance in

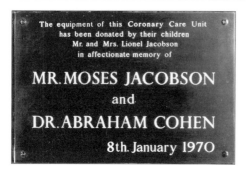

The equipment of this Coronary Care Unit
has been donated by their children
Mr. and Mrs. Lionel Jacobson
in affectionate memory of

MR. MOSES JACOBSON
and
DR. ABRAHAM COHEN

8th. January 1970

Plaque, formerly outside the Coronary Care Unit at the Newcastle General Hospital.

1966 and published with J. S. Geddes an account of it in *The Lancet* in 1967.[10] Immediately their results were published, Dewar set about starting a similar coronary ambulance in Newcastle. The Medical Officers of Health of Newcastle and of Northumberland, Drs Pearson and Tilley respectively, Mr William Collins, Assistant House Governor of the R.V.I. and Mr H. M. Roberts, Chief Ambulance Officer, were most helpful. The Regional Cardiovascular Unit at the General Hospital promised to cooperate.

Funded initially by a donation of £4,000 from the Jacobson Trust, and later by donations from patients and many well-wishers, it was organised by Drs John McCollum and Michael Floyd. It began operating in December 1967. An old ambulance was purchased from the NHS for £100, and fitted with special equipment. It was stationed at the R.V.I. and initially driven out by a doctor accompanied by a nurse, most often from the C.C.U. The ward sister, Rita Watkins, set an example by volunteering to take part. The doctors were also volunteers and all except one juniors, who at night slept in the hospital. They received no extra pay, but Lionel Jacobson again showed his generosity by donating funds for the salary of one full-time S.H.O. Dewar, who generated enthusiasm by taking part, remembers one of his first call-outs. The man lived in Byker, was about 70 years old, and was almost unconscious with a blood pressure of about 50 mm Hg. The E.C.G. showed myocardial infarction and over the next hour or so he slowly improved as his B.P. rose to about 90 mm Hg. When it was suggested to him that further recovery would be safer in the R.V.I., his reply was firm. 'A'm nae gannin tae that bloody place'. Nor did he, and he did well at home.

In this system, suggested by Dr Pearson, a second ambulance drove to the same address, the spare driver in it then bringing doctor, nurse and patient in the first vehicle back to the R.V.I., which at first had the only Coronary Care Unit. But doctors are not always good ambulance-drivers, and Dr Dewar had much sympathy with the excellent lady doctor who said to him that she had not supposed that, when she applied for a junior post in the R.V.I., she would be expected to drive a heavy ambulance, at night, and backwards, from its narrow parking place between two high walls! She wondered if a different system could be devised. Moreover, it proved only too easy for doctors, often unfamiliar with the city, to get lost.

Accordingly, after six months the procedure was altered to one in which the driver on duty at the ambulance centre came to the hospital to pick up the team and convey them quickly and reliably to the patient's address. There he waited to bring both team and patient back to whichever C.C.U. at either the R.V.I. or N.G.H. was on duty. An account of the first year of operation of the Newcastle Coronary Ambulance service was described in an article in the *British Medical Journal* in October 1969. [11] It demonstrated, as most other accounts have done, that the greatest delay, averaging 4½ hours from onset of a coronary thrombosis, occurs before the ambulance is called. Even then another 20 minutes passed before the medical team reached the patient. Provision of a new purposely built ambulance in 1969 greatly added to the comfort of the patient and the convenience of the nurse and doctor, but did little to reduce the delay in reaching the address. In 1973, once again, a new system was introduced, whereby the doctor and nurse and their equipment travelled in a 'minivan' direct to the patient, while an ambulance went independently to the same address. This halved the time, but the G.P.s still found it rather long, and analysis showed that the achievements of the unit were still unsatisfactory. Meanwhile, in 1971, Dr Douglas Chamberlain in Brighton had started training paramedics and in 1973 published greatly superior results. [12] Dewar, who with Dr Lawrence Bryson had visited him in Brighton, attempted to introduce his method into Newcastle. The young ambulance drivers were enthusiastic, the over-55s not surprisingly much less so, and the Chief Ambulance Officers in the two counties combined with the D.H.S.S. to render the change impossible. At the time of Dewar's retirement in 1978 the service was discontinued.

When, however, as is described in the chapter on research, there was introduced the 'fibrinolytic therapy' of coronary thrombosis, i.e. the means of actually dissolving the occluding clot by intravenous injection, it became more and more important that the patient should reach hospital really quickly. The treatment depends for its success entirely upon promptitude. More than six hours after onset of thrombosis, and it is useless. For this and other reasons, the excellent Chamberlain method of staffing emergency ambulances with paramedics was, after a few years of delay, finally accepted by the Ambulance Service. The men recruited are trained in both the Freeman Hospital and the R.V.I. The result is a conspicuous success. Each volunteer spends two weeks full-time in one or other of the coronary care units, to learn as much as possible about collapses, electrocardiograms, drugs, resuscitation techniques etc. and attends a refresher course every year thereafter. They work 12-hour shifts and receive some extra pay. The public certainly do not grudge it.

The chief objectives of such units, now established throughout the country, are: 1. to make a correct diagnosis, 2. to relieve pain and breathlessness, 3. to correct certain disturbances of heart rhythm, 4. to treat promptly and efficiently sudden stoppage of the heart, and, 5. (perhaps the most difficult task of all) to learn not to attempt to resuscitate the too late and hopeless. A heart which recovers when the brain will not is a disaster. Nor are relatives much comforted by futile attempts to revive a patient, dead for half an hour from a cerebral haemorrhage. The paramedics do not institute fibrinolytic treatment of the coronary thrombosis for the very good reason that the contra-indications are both numerous and dangerous. Because the R.V.I. lies in the centre of the city and provides the main Accident and Emergency Service for it, the majority of definite coronary thromboses are admitted to its C.C.U., while the Freeman, which is located towards the eastern edge, receives a high proportion of cases of 'unstable angina', (a kind of threatening thrombosis). The medical staff there are particularly interested in, and well equipped to deal with them. The paramedics have become skilful in making correct diagnoses, but the modern technique of transmitting an ECG by radio to cardiologists at base can be helpful in diagnosis of doubtful cases. Strangely, the greatest cause of delay still remains the reluctance of the Geordie to call for help when he develops a pain in his chest. Few cardiologists like to blame them too much, since their own record of making a correct diagnosis on themselves, when stricken, leaves them no excuse for pride!

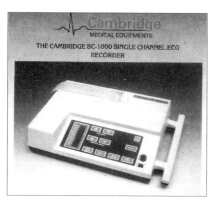

A modern Electrocardiograph 15½ × 10 × 3½ inches. Wt 7lbs.

All in all, the patient who today has a heart attack is more likely to survive it and be protected from having another one then ever seemed likely 40 years ago. The next advance ought to be the prevention of disease in the coronary arteries themselves. It is getting nearer.

Notes

1. Myers A., Dewar H. A., Circumstances attending 100 deaths from Coronary Artery Disease with Coroner's Necropsies. *Brit. Med. J.* 1975; 37: 1133–43.
2. Kouwenhoven W. B., Jude J. R., Knickerbocker G. G., Closed Chest Cardiac Massage. *J.A.M.A.* 1960; 173: 1064–7.
3. Kouwenhoven W. B., Milnor W. R., Treatment of Ventricular Fibrillation using Capacitor Discharge. *Appl. Physiol* 1954; 7: 253–57.
4. Lown B., Amarasingham R., Neuman J. New Method for Terminating Arrhythmias. *J.A.M.A.* 1962; 182: 548–55.
5. Julian D. G., Treatment of Cardiac Arrest in Acute Myocardial Ischaemia and Infarction. *Lancet* 1961; 2: 840–4.
6. Srivastava S. C., Dewar H. A., Newell D. J., Double-blind Trial of Propanolol (Inderal) in Angina of Effort. *Brit. Med. J.* 1964; 2: 724–5.
7. Reduction in Mortality after Myocardial Infarction with Long-term Beta-adrenergic blockade. A Multicentre International Study. *Brit. Med. J.* 1977; 2: 419–21.
8. Julian D. G., Prescott R. J., Jackson F. S., Szekely P., Controlled Trial of Sotalol for One Year after Myocardial Infarction. *Lancet* 1982; 1: (8282) 1142–7.
9. Dewar H. A., Advances in Cardiology, *Practitioner* 1965; 195: 449–55.
10. Pantridge J. F., Geddes J. S., A Mobile Intensive-care Unit in the Management of Myocardial Infarction. *Lancet* 1967; 2 (510): 271–3.
11. Dewar H. A., McCollum J. P. K., Floyd M., A Year's Experience with a Mobile Coronary Resuscitation Unit. *Brit. Med. J.* 1969; 4: 226–9.
12. White N. M., Parker W. S., Binning R. A., Kimber E. R., Ead H. W., Chamberlain D. A., *Brit. Med. J.* 1973; 3: 618–22.

CHAPTER 3

Implantable Pacemakers and Defibrillators

Pacemakers

In order to make the following account more intelligible to the non-medical reader, it is perhaps useful to outline the basic functions of a pacemaker. The tissue which conducts the impulse from the atria to the ventricles can be defective, a condition know as 'heart block'. The specialised tissue in the right atrium which is responsible for initiating the heartbeat may also be defective, resulting in a condition called 'sick sinus syndrome' or sinu-atrial block. In either case the effect is to produce a sudden and sometimes dramatic reduction or even cessation of the heartbeat, resulting in dizziness or loss of consciousness. To

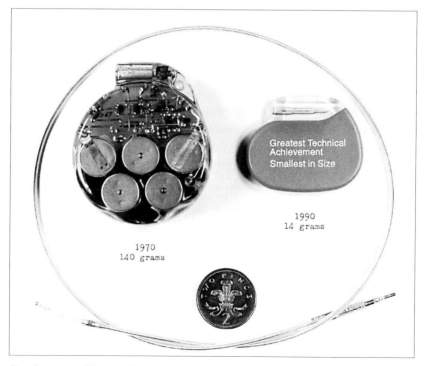

Development of Pacemakers.

remedy this, an artificial pacemaker is connected to the heart by a flexible insulated wire lead terminating in one or more electrodes. The lead is introduced into a vein either by exposing the cephalic vein near either shoulder, or nowadays commonly by percutaneous puncture of the subclavian vein below the collarbone with a needle. Depending on the nature of the abnormality, the electrode which conveys to the heart muscle the electrical stimulus generated by the pacemaker is embedded inside the apex of the right ventricle, or the right atrial appendage, or nowadays, often both. The other end of the lead or leads is connected to the pacemaker, which is a battery-powered device with the electrical circuitry to generate an impulse of the appropriate voltage and frequency and to sense what is happening to the patient's own heartbeat. The pacemaker is buried beneath the skin not far from the vein into which the wire is inserted. If for any reason this approach is unavailable or inappropriate, direct attachment of the electrode to the outside of the ventricle is used, and the pacemaker is then implanted in the upper abdominal wall.

The early pacemakers were large and because they used mercury\zinc batteries were also heavy, so that patients, especially the slim ones, were often conscious of the presence of the device under the skin. In this group, pacemaker extrusion was more likely to occur than in the large obese patient under whose skin and into whose deep layer of adipose tissue the pacemaker could easily be buried without a bulge.

The very first pacemakers had a fixed rate, usually about 70 beats per minute. However, as quite often the abnormality necessitating the use of a pacemaker is intermittent, a 'demand' type was soon devised. This was able to sense the patient's own heartbeat when it was present, and withhold its stimulus to avoid competition. Now not only these features but a number of others as well can be altered at the pacemaker follow-up clinic by an external 'programmer'. Indeed, many modern pacemakers can respond to the changing activity of the patient by increasing the pulse rate in response to exercise or by slowing it during the night.

Implantation of cardiac pacemakers began in the Northern Region in the mid-nineteen sixties. A few pacemakers were being implanted at both of the Regional Cardiothoracic Surgical Centres at Seaham Hall and Shotley Bridge, using the direct epicardial approach, but implantation via the transvenous route was confined initially to the Regional Cardio-vascular Department at Newcastle General Hospital and also at the Royal Victoria Infirmary, where the necessary cardiac catheterisation facilities were available. With the arrival of Dr Ronald Gold, implantation of cardiac pacemakers by the transvenous route was commenced at Shotley Bridge General Hospital in 1969. At both Newcastle General and Shotley Bridge a two-stage technique for implantation was used, in which the lead was introduced via the median cubital vein as an initial separate procedure. This had been devised by Gold and Paneth at the Brompton Hospital, but had been adopted in Newcastle before Gold's appointment there. In those early days, the rather primitive pacing leads were subject to a high rate of displacement during the first 24 hours. With a single-stage implantation, repositioning of the lead meant re-opening the pacemaker implantation site, with an increased risk of extrusion or infection. This could largely be avoided by delaying implantation of the pacemaker itself until 48 hours after insertion of the pacing lead. By this time late displacement was very uncommon. It also meant that implantation of the pacemaker itself could be carried out in a proper surgical environment, not available in the catheter laboratory at Newcastle General Hospital. During the next few years, with the special expertise available at Shotley Bridge, the number of patients being paced there increased rapidly, so that by the time the Cardiothoracic Unit moved to Freeman Hospital in 1977, Shotley Bridge had become the major implanting centre in the region. In the early days the policy was to reposition a displaced transvenous electrode on one occasion only, because of the increased risk of sepsis. If a subsequent further displacement occurred, the pacemaker would be implanted by the epicardial approach. This required the services of a cardiothoracic surgeon, so that the patients paced at Shotley Bridge included a number of patients from the other hospital when transvenous electrodes had become displaced.

Because of its relative inaccessibility geographically, only patients living locally attended Shotley Bridge for their follow-up pacemaker checks and the largest pacemaker follow-up clinic was at Newcastle General Hospital. The increasing numbers of pacemaker patients requiring follow-up resulted in an expansion in the number and frequency of pacemaker clinics. With the opening of Freeman Hospital, the pacemaker clinics already in existence at Newcastle General Hospital and Shotley Bridge moved there. Clinics were established at Darlington Memorial Hospital and Cumberland Infirmary, Carlisle, initially using a telephone link to the Regional Pacing Department at Freeman Hospital, which enabled pacemaker function tests to be carried out over the telephone line by the technician at Freeman Hospital. This evoked quite a lot of media attention and the first transmission from Carlisle was filmed by both the BBC and ITV for their local news services. A few weeks later BBC's 'Tomorrow's World' included a live telecast of a trans-telephonic transmission from a pacemaker patient in their studios in London to Freeman Hospital. The resulting ECG recording at Freeman Hospital, when compared subsequently with that taken directly from the patient, was indistinguishable. Telephone lines were not, however, always as good as the BBC managed to obtain. The technique worked well at Carlisle, where Dr Howard Robson had been appointed as a Consultant Physician with a specialist interest in Cardiology, and remained in use for several years. A formal evaluation of the technique and the apparatus and its cost-effectiveness was carried out by Gold and his team for the Department of Health. A similar attempt to link Darlington Memorial Hospital with the Freeman Hospital proved unsuccessful because of the then lack of the necessary cardiological and technical expertise there. This was remedied by regular visits to Darlington by Gold and an experienced cardiac technician.

The pacemakers of the nineteen-sixties were very primitive by today's standards. The earliest fixed rate models had no sensing capabilities. This resulted in frequent competition between the pacemaker and the patient's intrinsic heart rhythm, but ventricular fibrillation from the 'R on T' phenomenon was extremely uncommon. Later models were of the 'demand' type but their life span was short, often less than three years. All pacemakers of that era were of the single-chamber ventricular pacing type and even when, in the early 'seventies, atrially triggered ventricular pacing units became available, their cost was too high for their routine use. The anti-tachycardia functions which are now frequently incorporated in pacemakers, and pacemakers designed primarily for the treatment of tachycardias, were quite unheard of in those days.

The most dramatic advance in pacemaker technology was the development of the lithium battery as a power source. This resulted in much smaller pacemakers as much of the bulk of the earlier units was due to the four or five mercury-zinc cells necessary to power them. This greatly facilitated the pacing of young children, in whom previously the pacemakers, because of their large size, were often implanted inside the rib cage. The mercury-zinc cells also had the disadvantage that they produced hydrogen gas as they aged, and this accumulated under pressure in the sealed epoxy resin case of the pacemaker. On one occasion at Shotley Bridge, removal of such a pacemaker from a patient who had kept his routine appointment at the pacemaker clinic, where evidence of battery depletion had been found, revealed that a small explosion had occurred, cracking the epoxy case. On questioning, the patient did admit to feeling 'a bit of a thump over the pacemaker a few weeks ago'! Programmable pacemakers, now so much taken for granted, were also initially too expensive for routine use, as were the later dual-chamber physiological pacemakers, now recommended by the British Pacing and Electrophysiology Group for routine use. The increased financial burden of adopting these recommendations was the subject of a published study carried out in the Regional Pacing Centre at Freeman Hospital. Although it is difficult to compare like with like, pacemakers have actually become cheaper over the years. In 1968 one paid £255 for a simple non-programmable single chamber 'demand' pacemaker, whereas twenty years later a model with similar rudimentary specifications, but likely to last three times as long, cost only double that amount.

With the tremendous advances in pacemaker technology over the past two decades and the reliability of pacemaker systems today, it is hard to remember the trials and tribulations, but also the excitement and sense of achievement involved, for both patient and doctor in those early days of pacing. Hopefully this account will at least in part redress this.

Implantable Defibrillators

In the chapter on the prevention and treatment of heart attacks an account has been given of how the most dangerous, and if uncorrected, fatal type of disturbed rhythm of the heart, ventricular fibrillation (VF), can be terminated by a high voltage electric shock applied externally by two large electrodes placed on the front of the chest. In some patients these attacks are recurrent and cannot be suppressed by drug treatment. If they are not immediately detected and treated, death is inevitable. In the 1970s a defibrillator was devised, similar in operation to the external defibrillator but small enough to be implanted in the patient and incorporating a means of monitoring the patient's ECG to detect the onset of VF. During the 1980s the use of this apparatus in humans became a realistic proposition, although the very high cost of the apparatus, around £10,000, was a severe deterrent to its use except in the most desperate cases. The first such device in Newcastle was implanted in 1989 (?) at Freeman Hospital.

In those days, in addition to a transvenous electrode similar to, but much larger than, those used for pacing, a large wire mesh electrode had to be stitched to the outside of the heart, thus involving the need for the chest to be opened and the electrode placed in position by a cardiac surgeon. Furthermore, the defibrillator itself was huge, about twice the size of the largest early pacemaker, and this posed problems with the siting of the unit, especially in the thin patient.

A major problem in those early days was the correct identification by the defibrillator of the presence of ventricular fibrillation, so that it was not uncommon for the defibrillator to discharge inappropriately. The large amount of electrical energy at that time needed for the procedure to be effective meant a very limited battery life of the unit, still further shortened when inappropriate discharges were frequent. Nowadays, the electrical energy required for successful defibrillation is much less, so that the defibrillator has become much smaller, despite it also incorporating a number of other features such as the ability to pace the heart for bradycardia, as described in the first part of this chapter, and various antitachycardia functions enabling it to terminate rhythm disturbances other than ventricular fibrillation. The electrodes for defibrillation can now be inserted tranvenously and the whole procedure carried out by a cardiologist, without the need for the chest to be opened. Where drug treatment and surgery as described in the chapter on research fail to control life-threatening disturbances of cardiac rhythm, the implantable defibrillator is now a realistic and practical alternative. An increasing number of patients in the region owe their very survival to the device and regard the inconvenience and discomfort of being defibrillated, even if still occasionally inappropriately, as a small price to pay for this.

CHAPTER 4

PAEDIATRIC CARDIOLOGY

In the years preceding the introduction of antibiotics, rheumatic fever and chorea were very common maladies in childhood and responsible for a high proportion of the cases of valvular heart disease which were encountered in adolescence and adult life. Toxic myocarditis was the principal cause of death when children developed diphtheria, and if bacterial endocarditis complicated rheumatic or congenital heart disease, it was invariably fatal. All these maladies were particularly prevalent in the North East, where poverty, malnutrition and over-crowding were important contributing factors. Congenital malformations were presumably also very common and, since no surgical treatment was available, very often fatal. French physicians such as Fallot and Roger had made the clinical features of some of them recognisable, and the Canadian physician Maud Abbott's atlas, published in 1936, systematised much of the knowledge available. Sir James Mackenzie (1853–1925), by correlating his polygraph tracings with observations of how patients fared over the years, had ensured that young people with sinus arrhythmia or a few 'extra-systoles' were not put to bed for months on end. The part played by viruses in causing heart problems was unrecognised, to begin with because viruses were unknown and later because they were thought to be unimportant.

Paediatrics as a speciality did not exist and children who needed to be in hospital for diagnosis or treatment would be cared for by consultant physicians in the children's wards of the R.V.I., and in the Fleming Memorial Hospital for Sick Children, or in the Infectious Diseases Hospital by general practitioners and hospital doctors. As already described, Hume took an interest in his early years in the dysrhythmias of diphtheritic myocarditis and correlated them with the pathological changes found in the heart at post mortem. He also became expert in the use of the only anti-dysrhythmic drugs available – digitalis and quinidine – and the only medicament available for active rheumatism, sodium salicylate. In the years immediately preceding the Second World War, clinical instruction of medical students in paediatrics was in the hands of Dr James Lickley, a general practitioner erudite in anatomy and neurology and a capable and experienced, if rather uninspiring, teacher. Only when he retired during that war, did James Spence, hitherto a general physician, take over paediatrics and establish what became a world-famous department.

After the war everything changed. The discovery of antibiotics and an enormous improvement in anaesthesia allowed surgery to be undertaken for both congenital malformations and rheumatic valvular heart disease. With universal immunisation, diphtheria virtually disappeared. Both Swan's team at the N.G.H. and presently Henderson at Shotley Bridge, and simultaneously Dewar at the R.V.I., undertook investigation of the cases prior to surgical treatment. For some of the defects, such as a patent ductus arteriosus, special investigations were not needed, although occasionally insisted upon by the surgeon, but for many others they were necessary in order to assess the full severity or to exclude abnormalities such as significant valvular regurgitation or the kind of atrial septal defect which would make 'closed' surgical operations or operation under hypothermia rather than under cardiopulmonary by-pass (a later development) unsuitable.

For all of these the chief link with paediatrics was Marion Bethune. After a brilliant undergraduate career, followed by experience in both cardiology and paediatrics in Edinburgh and Southampton, in 1952 she was appointed paediatric registrar to the R.V.I., the N.G.H. and the Babies Hospital in Newcastle. From the outset, her skill in the diagnosis and management of all forms of heart disease in children was appreciated by the cardiologists Swan, Henderson and Dewar, with whom she worked. From the latter two she learned, and rather infrequently practised, the techniques of cardiac catheterisation and angiography. The delay in her

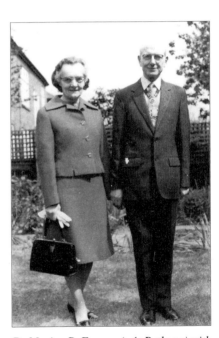

Dr Marion B. Farmer (née Bethune) with her husband Frank (Frank T. Farmer, Professor of Medical Physics) M.D. (Ed.), F.R.C.P.E., D.C.H., Consultant Paediatrician, Babies Hospital, R.V.I., N.G.H. and Freeman Hospitals, 1966–74.

promotion to consultant status in 1966 from senior registrar (1954) was due to administrative difficulties, not lack of support by her colleagues. She got through an extraordinary amount of work in the three hospitals mentioned, as well as at Shotley Bridge, which was added to her remit in 1957. Yet she still found time to visit cardiological clinics at the Hammersmith Hospital and Great Ormond Street and, in 1962, similar clinics in North America. A skilled diagnostician, probably her most valued strength lay in gaining the confidence and affection of parents and children, so that they trusted her implicitly and felt, after she had talked to them, that they understood the technical problem as completely as was possible for a lay person. They also knew that she would be the child's doctor before, during and long after, any operation.

Her liaison with other paediatric surgical centres in the U.K. was particularly valuable because, although the surgical unit at Shotley Bridge started operating on hearts quite early and kept abreast of new developments, it did not at first attain, especially for more difficult cases, the excellent results with low mortality which similar clinics achieved elsewhere. In the meantime a substantial proportion of the children who needed operations were sent by Marion Bethune and the cardiologists to other centres, especially in London.

The risks of surgical treatment of children, however, decreased considerably when, in 1961, Mr Selwyn Griffin and his team began operating at Seaham Hall as a separate unit, as is described in the chapter on Surgery, though he had been operating there part-time for a few years and ligatured a patent ductus in 1956. But the greatest progress toward a first-class surgical service for congenital heart disease came with the appointment in 1966 of Mr Ary Blesovsky and in 1974 of Mr Michael Holden. Ligation of ducts, resection of coarctation of the aorta and correction of atrial and ventricular septal defects had been carried out, as we have seen, since the early 1960s, but with the arrival of Ary Blesovsky correction of the more serious lesions such as Tetralogy of Fallot took off. The cardiological cover at this stage was less well defined and fell heavily on the shoulders of two people, Marion Farmer (née Bethune; she had married Frank Farmer, Professor of Medical Physics in 1960) and Charles Henderson. These two individuals brought their particular skills to the management of congenital heart disease. Charles Henderson was a remarkably adept investigator and catheteriser who enjoyed solving problems. Marion Farmer's invaluable qualities as primarily a paediatrician have already been discussed. Together based at the cardiology department of Newcastle General Hospital and at the Babies Hospital, they set up a service for congenital heart disease which linked the developing department of cardiology and the already prestigious paediatric department of Professor Donald Court (successor to Sir James Spence).

Until the appointment of Dr Ronald Gold in 1967, Charles Henderson was the only cardiologist in the region with specific expertise in performing cardiac catheterisation in young children. He visited Shotley Bridge periodically and carried out some catheterisations there but the value of these procedures was considerably limited by the primitive equipment then available in the catheter laboratory there. Ronald Gold had had extensive training and experience in the catheterisation of patients of all ages with congenital heart disease during his time at the Brompton Hospital in London and, with his arrival and the upgrading of the catheterisation facilities at Shotley Bridge, he was able to perform his own investigations on the quite numerous young children referred to his clinics, particularly at Darlington and Bishop Auckland, by the paediatricians. He retained his interest in congenital heart disease even after the opening of Freeman Hospital, but selectively referred the more complicated cases to his paediatric cardiologist colleagues.

In the early days, following the example set at Great Ormond Street Hospital in London and at the Toronto Children's Hospital, cardiac catheterisation of children was performed under local anaesthesia using some sedation. While at the Brompton Hospital, Gold carried out all his catheterisation on such patients under general anaesthesia with controlled ventilation, which produced a much steadier haemodynamic state than in the often very restless, or alternatively over-sedated and sometimes mildly hypoxic, unanaesthetised patient. At Shotley Bridge, with the help and skilled anaesthetic support of Dr Derek Pearson, he was able to develop these techniques further, in particular the use of routine monitoring of blood gases during the procedure. They were able to convince their initially sceptical paediatric cardiological colleagues, so that general anaesthesia became routine in the catheterisation of babies and young children.

During this period a major spurt in technology and expertise occurred in paediatric cardiology. Professor Senning and Dr Mustard, in different parts of the Western world, contrived new operations for dealing with transposition of the great arteries and in the United States Dr Bill Rashkind introduced a remarkable life-saving device called the balloon atrial septostomy catheter. Suddenly more children were surviving with serious congenital heart disease and the workload, not for the last time in paediatric cardiology, mushroomed.

The first two people appointed specifically to deal with congenital heart disease were Dr Stewart Hunter and Dr Michael Tynan. Stewart was in post as a Research Fellow in paediatric cardiology from 1969 and Michael, who came from Great Ormond Street Hospital and was one of the most innovative of the then new breed of young paediatric cardiologists, was appointed as consultant in 1971. Stewart went as a Research Fellow to Pennsylvania State University in 1972, and in 1973 returned to Newcastle as the second consultant on what was to become a flourishing Department of Paediatric Cardiology. For the first time there were people who were trained specifically as paediatric cardiologists to look after congenital heart disease as a sole occupation, rather than as a paediatrician or adult cardiologist with a special interest.

The department at the General Hospital blossomed and grew. A new technological wonder arrived in the shape of cardiac ultrasound or echocardiography. In Newcastle, as in many other centres, the introduction of the technique was by paediatric cardiologists who were most practised in its use. From the early seventies onwards, Newcastle acquired, and still retains, an international reputation for its 'Recent advances and training' echocardiography course. The course covered all aspects of cardiac ultrasound, gradually increasing its scope so that it now covers foetal diagnosis, intraoperative diagnosis, transoesophageal diagnosis and exercise echocardiography. There are now many training courses in echocardiography throughout Europe but Newcastle's was the first.

After a few years in Newcastle, the ever-stimulating Michael Tynan was lured back to his roots and became first of all consultant cardiologist at Guy's Hospital and subsequently achieved a Chair in paediatric cardiology at that institution. In his place came Hugh Bain, an Edinburgh graduate, trained in Toronto and Leeds.

It was obvious to the cardiologists and surgeons of Newcastle that the service to cardiological patients was ludicrously spread out.

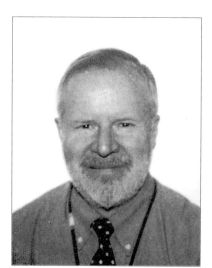

Dr. A. Stewart Hunter M.B., Ch.B. (Aberd.), F.R.C.P. (Ed. and Glas.), D.C.H., Consultant Paediatric Cardiologist, Freeman Hospital, Newcastle.

The opportunity of a new teaching hospital at Freeman Road was grasped eagerly to bring together all the disparate skills and clinical needs in a regional cardiothoracic department amid the woods and fields of Heaton. Paediatric cardiology continued to develop in this new venue. The two cardiologists became ever more involved in an enlarging and increasingly successful practice. Paediatric anaesthetists skilled in managing congenital heart disease were sought and found. A new Children's Intensive Care Unit was provided courtesy of the Children's Heart Unit Fund, a registered charity supporting paediatric cardiology in the Northern region. Close links with the Academic Department of Cardiology, first of all under Desmond Julian and then under Ronnie Campbell, were maintained and in due course, again funded by the Children's Heart Unit Fund. Christopher Wren joined the department, initially as a senior registrar and subsequently as the third paediatric cardiological consultant. Ary Blesovsky retired and Mike Holden, for reasons of health, had to give up the surgical care of small children and there was a difficult time for a year or two when the department existed on 'mail order surgery' provided by surgeons coming from Great Ormond Street weekly. However, eventually the department was able to attract Leslie Hamilton, an Ulsterman with Canadian connections and trained in Leeds, to come and head up the surgical side of congenital heart disease. More recently Asif Hasan joined as second surgeon, with a strong interest in congenital heart disease. The management of congenital heart disease is now very complex and covers the foetus, the neonate, the infant, the adolescent and the adult. The surgical advances in the last few years associated with the new speciality of interventional cardiology, have continued to push forward the frontiers. The treatment of congenital heart disease has benefited enormously by being associated with the main cardiothoracic centre, first of all at Newcastle General Hospital, then at Freeman Hospital. The mingling of clinical expertise and the sharing of costly facilities has ensured that the congenital heart disease patients in the North East continue to have a quality of care which is unsurpassed in the United Kingdom. It would, of course, be wrong to finish without pointing out that the department of paediatric cardiology and surgery at Freeman is one of three units in the country designated for children's heart and heart/lung transplantation and to ponder a future where small children with severely malformed hearts may benefit from transplants, courtesy of transgenic pigs farmed at the back of the hospital site. It could happen.

CHAPTER 5

RESEARCH

Research on cardiology, like everything else on the subject in New-castle, began with Hume. Sir James Mackenzie had Marey's poly-graph adapted, exchanging the smoked drum for an ink pen, and had demonstrated that, by using the instrument to distinguish between sinus arrhythmia, the different types of 'extra systoles' and atrial fibrillation, and combining the observation with many years of follow-up of the patients, one could distinguish between the always harmless, the some-times dangerous and the always sinister. [1] Hume spent many hours in the wards of the infectious diseases hospital studying the very varied dis-turbances of rhythm which occurred in the myocarditis of diphtheria, a disease both common and dangerous in those days. He published his findings in the new journal *Heart*, of which Sir Thomas Lewis was founder and editor. Another of these contributions, as already noted, was one of the early accounts of atrial flutter. [2] During the First World War and subsequently in civilian life, he made useful contributions to medical literature on the myocarditis of spirochaetal jaundice, a dangerous ma-lady contracted from rats in the trenches of Northern France and in the coal mines of North East England. His Bradshaw Lecture at the Royal College of Physicians was on paroxysmal tachycardia. Between the two wars, however, the need to provide for his wife and family wholly from private practice and his many other commitments rendered it impossible for him to conduct much research himself, and the meagre staffing – one house physician and one registrar shared with the Assistant Physician – afforded little opportunity to stimulate others.

One interesting but unsuccessful piece of research was accomplished by Laurence O'Shaughnessy shortly before the Second World War, in the first year of which, sadly, he was killed. He was a Durham graduate who had passed his M.B. B.S. examination at 21 years of age and the F.R.C.S. at 23. Impressed with the extensive anastomoses (alternative channels) which developed around the abdominal omentum (a fatty kind of apron, enclosing part of the gut) in cases of cirrhosis of the liver, and which conveyed into the systemic blood stream so much of what could no longer traverse the liver, he conceived the idea that the omentum, if applied to the surface of an ischaemic heart, might provide an alternative blood supply just where it was needed. Experimental work on greyhounds supported the concept and in 1938 he persuaded George Mason, who was already doing thoracic surgery, to undertake cardio-omentopexy. The patient who improved most, becoming angina-free, unkindly died later. Autopsy showed one anastomotic vessel, of the calibre of cotton thread. The occasional tendency of angina to improve spontaneously has deceived many a research worker before and since.

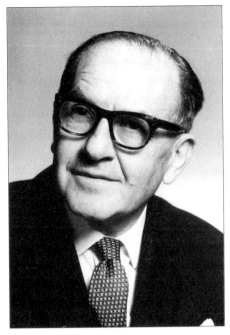

Dr Paul Szekely M.D. (Prague), F.R.C.P. (London), Consultant Cardiologist, Newcastle General Hospital, 1948–75.

The introduction of the National Health Service in 1948 gave a tremendous fillip to research. Relieved of the need to earn their living solely from private practice, and with more generous staffing by juniors, consultants were able to plan and initiate research projects in which doctors in training were able to play major or minor parts. Paul Szekely, who had published his first paper on electro-cardiography within three years of qualifying in medicine in Prague, joined Hume in 1941 at the Newcastle General Hospital, first as house physician, later becoming registrar and consultant. Between 1941 and 1968 he published more than 40 papers. They covered a wide range of topics – cardiac involvement in spirochaetal jaundice (with Hume), cardiac pharmacology, *viz* the effects on the heart of magnesium, calcium, digitalis, procaine and propranolol, cardioversion, hypothermia and pulmonary embolism. The two subjects on which his international reputation stood highest were rheumatic fever, with its cardiological consequences, and heart disease in pregnancy. His articles in joint authorship with his obstetrical colleague Linton Snaith on 'The Heart in Toxaemia of Pregnancy' [3] and 'The Place of Cardiac Surgery in the Management of the Pregnant Woman with Heart Disease' [4] were the forerunners of their classical text book on the subject, *Heart Disease and Pregnancy*,[5] which was to appear in 1974. Fluent in five languages and an indefatigable attender and speaker at cardiological meetings world-wide, no cardiologist in Newcastle, until the arrival of Professor Julian, attained during those post-war years so high an international reputation.

Adrian Swan, an excellent clinical cardiologist and a good teacher of students, published little, his best paper probably being a perceptive account of 'Acute Non-Specific Pericarditis',[6] His long association with the Venereal Disease Unit at the Newcastle General Hospital made him an expert on the cardiovascular effects of syphilis. He collaborated with Dewar in a paper on the heart in haemochromatosis.[7] Marion Bethune (later Mrs Farmer) wrote her M.D. thesis on patent ductus arteriosus, of which she had experience of 110 cases, 70 of them submitted to oper-ation. She also contributed a section on heart disease to Professor Court's book on *The Medical Care of Children*[8] and collaborated with Paul Szekely in a paper on 'Rheumatic Fever and Rheumatic Heart Disease – Natural History and Preventive Aspects'.[9] Her paper in the *Newcastle Medical Journal* in 1958 on 'General Care of a Child with Congenital Heart Disease' was a distillation of her great experience and sympathetic devotion.

Meanwhile at the Royal Victoria Infirmary Hewan Dewar, having co-operated with Ian Hill in a paper on effort syndrome,[10] had in 1947 been appointed as Assistant Physician, largely on the strength of some research, never published, on myasthenia gravis, which he had begun in 1946. There was great interest at that time in this disease, which is characterised by profound weakness of muscles in response to exercise and by a puzzling enlargement of the thymus gland. Removal of the gland sometimes led to substantial improvement. As soon as he learned the use of cardiac catheters, he and Tommy Grimson, later Consultant Physician at Chester-le-Street, arranged with George Mason to direct one into the thymic vein of a case of myasthenia gravis whose thymus Mason had been asked by Professor Nattrass to excise. The blood withdrawn was then applied to the neuromuscular preparation of a frog which Dewar and Grimson had prepared in the Medical School and conveyed by car to Shotley Bridge. No paralysing effect ensued and so ended a project which was imaginative, logical and wholly futile. However, over the 20 years between 1948 and 1968, Dewar, in collaboration with numerous other gifted assistants, published some 38 papers on anti-anginal and anti-hypertensive drug trials, cerebral blood flow in mitral stenosis and, in 1961, the first of a series of papers on fibrinolysis *viz* 'Fibrinolytic

Treatment of Coronary Thrombosis – a Pilot Study'. [11] This was followed in 1963 by a proper controlled trial in which the 'Thrombolysis' was compared with glucose in saline in 75 cases of acute coronary thrombosis treated within a mean of 6.2 hours of onset (range 3–12) and the results were wholly negative. [12] This was probably because the medicament, claimed by its manufacturer to be plasmin but widely believed to be streptokinase, really was plasmin, and therefore, as was later recognised, promptly destroyed in the bloodstream. To be effective Streptokinase must activate its precursor plasminogen, which has already become absorbed into the fibrin in the clot. The plasmin then dissolves it. In this work on fibrinolysis a most important part was played by I. Sudhakaran Menon, a very capable and enterprising Indian graduate. Over some four years, culminating in a Newcastle Ph.D., he initiated and collaborated in a series of experiments and trials. Several of his papers were concerned with the fibrinolytic activity (FA) in the venous effluent of different organs of the body. Other interesting topics were the demonstration that the clinical variations of FA and cortisol, though inverse, were unlikely to be causally related, and that the veins of the paralysed limb of a hemiplegic patient display increased rather then decreased FA. [13] This may explain why embolism from such a limb is infrequent.

In 1969 Dewar and Menon were invited to take part in an internationally organised trial of streptokinase in comparison with heparin. [14] In this series the mean time elapsing from onset of symptoms to initiation of treatment was much longer, 20 hours, and this may well have been an important factor in its also negative result. But Dewar maintained his belief that streptokinase (SK) had a future as a therapeutic agent, for both peripheral vascular

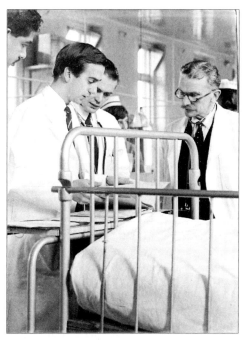

From left to right: Drs I.S. Menon, Jeremy Fegetter, Roger White, and Hewan Dewar.

and coronary occlusion, and in 1976–77 with the help of R. H. Smith, expert in coronary catheterisation, and P. Hacking, radiologist, treated six cases of the latter with intra-coronary infusions. The object was to prove that lysis of such thrombi could indeed take place. The best result obtained in the experiment is shown in the accompanying angiographic plate. In 1977 the full results were demonstrated both to a joint meeting of the British and Swedish Cardiac Societies (recorded in the *British Heart Journal* 1978) and to a meeting of the International Society of Fibrinolysis. Neither showed much interest. The *British Medical Journal* declined to publish the report as being too specialised and the *American Journal of Cardiology* found it faultless but of too little interest for any priority. It was finally published in the *Proceedings of the International Society on Fibrinolysis*, Vol IV, pp. 273–9.

Fortunately a German, P. Rentrop, conceived the same idea and in 1980, after trying intracoronary SK on a single case a few months before, published with colleagues in 1980 in *Dtsch. Med. Wschr.*; 105(7): 221–8 a series of 6 cases of primary coronary thrombosis, in whom recanalisation could be demonstrated. They followed it a year later (*Amer. Heart J.*; 102 (6PT.2): 1181–7) by a series of 204 patients in whom infusion of SK, still by the intracoronary route, achieved a 60% success in recanalisation with much reduced mortality. Since then numerous trials have shown that intravenous use of the drug, a considerably more practical, though perhaps less efficacious, method, will indeed reduce mortality. It is now used world-wide as a routine procedure for suitable patients. Dewar himself retired early in 1978. His last contribution on the subject of coronary lysis was a short publication with his successor Roger Hall showing that while prostacyclin, a potent arterial dilator and platelet disaggregator, might or might not be of clinical value in the treatment of an acute coronary occlusion, its intracoronary infusion was at least harmless. [15]

In Newcastle the fibrinolytic treatment of coronary thrombosis began in the Freeman Hospital routinely in 1986, but the unit had been active before that by taking part in international trials, as described below. Initially, following Rentrop's lead, the drug was given by direct injection

---

Opposite: *Demonstration by Drs H.A. Dewar, R.H. Smith and P.M. Hacking in 1976–7 of lysis (dissolution) of thrombi by direct injection of streptokinase through a cardiac catheter into a coronary artery. Explanatory drawings by Dr R.A.L. Brewis.*
Top: *Thrombus in anterior descending branch of L. coronary artery.*
Bottom: *Thrombus (embolic?) in circumflex branch of L. coronary artery. Artificial (prosthetic) aortic and mitral valves present.*

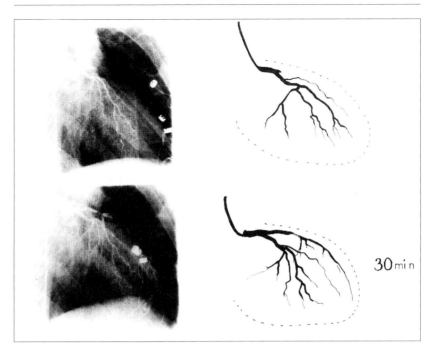

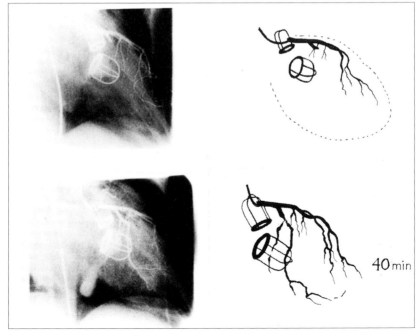

into the occluded coronary artery, but later this was changed to the intravenous route, as had been the practice in the earlier 'thrombolysin' trials. The proper purpose of giving it directly into the coronary artery, as Dewar had intended in 1977 and Rentrop had come to appreciate, was to show that the drug really did work. Later research, some of it undertaken in Newcastle (vide footnote), has been to demonstrate by other means (changes in ECG's and cardiac enzymes) that the treatment had indeed salvaged heart muscle. [16]

With the arrival of Professor Julian in 1975, research received a tremendous boost, and then a second one when in 1986 Professor Campbell succeeded to his place. Fertile with ideas, well funded by the British Heart Foundation (B.H.F.) and able to select gifted research assistants, each has been able to present back to the parent body a list of high quality research papers. These in a decade have exceeded in number what previous investigators have produced in a working lifetime! The historian can do no more than indicate broadly the various areas in which advances have been made. The full list is, of course, available through Medline under the subject headings and, through their titles, the names of the many colleagues and assistants who have done so much of the investigative work in this new and congenial academic environment.

The following are the main areas in which research has been conducted:

1. (a) After Rentrop's demonstration that coronary thrombi could indeed be dissolved, a number of international trials were started to establish whether such treatment would reduced mortality without serious risk of haemorrhage into the brain, the damaged heart muscle or elsewhere. Answers were also sought to questions such as optimal dosage, best drugs to prevent recurrence of thrombosis, and how one can detect and assess salvage. There had also for many years been available three different forms of lytic agent, one 2½ and another 8 times more expensive than the cheapest. There can be good reasons for prescribing the latter but they needed to be made clear. Taking into account the high standing of Julian's department, one is not surprised that all the cardiac departments in the Newcastle Teaching Hospitals were invited to take part in these trials. His own skill in summarising and evaluating the results are shown in several published papers. The routine use of fibrinolytic treatment for coronary thrombosis in Newcastle began in 1986.

Incidental to the above have also been some studies of the place of a

Beta-blocking drug (sotalol) and of ACE inhibitors in the management of the infarct patient. [17,18]

(b) Soon after arriving in Newcastle as First Assistant to Julian, Campbell began, with the indispensable co-operation of Newcastle University's Department of Medical Physics, those studies of the disturbances of the rhythm of the heartbeat which have made the Newcastle Medical School famous throughout the world. In this connection it is interesting that Hume, in 1930, gave the Bradshaw Lecture of the Royal College of Physicians on 'The Paroxysmal Tachycardias'. In 1971 Julian gave the same eponymous lecture on 'The Significance and Management of Ventricular Arrhythmias', a not very different title. The latter brought out the tremendous advances which have been made in our understanding of the subject in the intervening years, especially in the last two decades. Hume studied the ECG, as recorded by electrodes placed on both wrists and one ankle. Julian's team studied it as recorded by a needle electrode placed very precisely in different 'pin-point' areas inside the heart itself. The reasons for doing so are relevant to both the acute coronary situation and to patients prone to attacks of Ventricular Tachycardia (VT) and sometimes of Fibrillation (VF), arising from less urgent coronary disease or a variety of other maladies of the heart.

(c) Measurements of Q-T Dispersion can in some instances 'non-invasively' achieve the same result. It had been noted that sometimes in a patient the Q-T interval (the duration of repolarisation or recovery of muscle after contraction) varied between the ECG leads, i.e. between different areas of the heart. The amount of this variation is related to the risk of arrhythmias.

The object in all cases has been to provide prediction and prevention. When drugs fail, then more radical methods are required. Some striking successes have been achieved. First it was found that in most cases of recurrent VT the focus, often a quite small group of muscle fibres, could by investigation be identified. The next step was to ask a surgeon to remove it. This, of course, meant an 'open-heart' operation, but despite the obvious risks, 150 were successfully so treated without a single death, a tribute to the skill of Janet McComb and Colin Hilton. It is no wonder that the cardiac department attracted research workers from this and several other countries to learn the technique, and that cases were sent to it from all over the region for investigation and treatment. Not surprisingly, Professor Campbell was invited to give lectures on the subject all over the world, and most prestigiously in 1990 gave the Darwin Lecture to the British Association for the Advancement of Science. Most happily for patients, the later discovery elsewhere that the same curative effect could be obtained by a laser introduced through a catheter in an artery has rendered the operation obsolete and this laser treatment is now routine procedure in the Newcastle Department. But precise identification of the focus remains a skilled and essential task. If the procedure fails or is impossible, an automatic defibrillator is implanted.

(d) A team of Newcastle cardiologists, neurologists and an anaesthetist has investigated the amount of harm to the brain which can arise during cardiopulmonary bypass operations for relief or cure of coronary heart disease, and the reasons for it. Despite every precaution, it is probably impossible to prevent harm totally, but the long term findings are reassuring.

(e) Co-operation with Professor Oliver James, a long-time student of liver disease, has enlarged understanding of the damage to the heart which can follow from chronic alcoholism.

(f) An interesting and important study by two cardiologists and a Professor of Medicine has shed some more light on the extremely complex problem of the interaction of heredity, diet, and blood proteins in the development of coronary artery disease.

2. In the paediatric field new techniques, especially that of echocardiography, were developed, leading to important advances in knowledge. These advances can be grouped into:

(a) Studies into how, by placing the echotransmitter on to new sites, such as just beyond the upper and lower ends of the sternum (breast bone), and sometimes in two planes at once, many of the extraordinarily complicated and varied congenital malformations encountered can be detected early in life and even before birth. Not only is their existence detected, but also precise anatomical details. As a refinement, this use of ultrasound can be combined with the 'Doppler' method of measuring bloodflow to measure pressures also. This is of particular importance, since high pressures in the pulmonary bloodvessels lead in time to irreversible and serious changes in them. In other words, the degree of urgency for surgical correction can be assessed as well as the possibility of surgery at all.

The need for 'invasive' methods of investigation – catheterisation and angiography – in children has not been eliminated, but use of them can often be delayed. In any case, the combination of all three methods often provides more information than would the use of only two. A number of the published papers concern this theme.

(b) The Haemodyamics of Pregnancy. The unit has, in combination with the Department of Obstetrics, used Echo and Doppler in a very important study of the haemodyamics of normal pregnancy. No one would wish to use cardiac catheterisation or angiography on a pregnant woman unless it was absolutely necessary. Echocardiography appears to be totally harmless and is certainly not unpleasant. It has, therefore, been possible to determine, as pregnancy proceeds, how bloodflow through the lungs increases, how their small arterioles relax to accommodate it without any rise in pressure, and how the heart responds to the increased work, much as those of athletes do! To know the normal is invaluable when one meets the abnormal. For the first time the normal parameters are firmly established. The study even extended to normal breast feeding.

As a side-issue, making use of the department's expertise in the technique, a study was made with Dr R. J. C. Hall, then cardiologist at the R.V.I., of how, by echocardiography, the severity of a valve defect (mitral stenosis) can be assessed. Once again X-ray exposure was avoided.

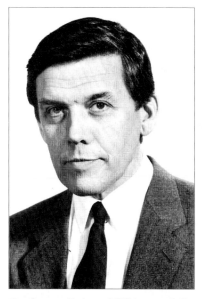

(c) Heart transplants in children. The benefits which can now follow from early diagnosis (before, at, or soon after birth) and operation upon serious heart malformations have been described (22 transplants between 1985 and 1992 with only two deaths). A survey made showed that the call for transplants is not likely to diminish. Sadly or fortunately, depending on how one

Professor Robert Wilkinson B.Sc. (Durham) MD., F.R.C.P., Professor of Renal Medicine, University of Newcastle

looks at it, the opportunities for such a procedure are never likely to match the need. One other valuable joint study has shown that it is possible to establish a regime of anti-rejection treatment by drugs with only a small amount of steroids in them. Thus retardation of growth can be minimised.

(d) Genetics. Since congenital malformations cannot always be totally corrected, and they are in any case very undesirable, a beginning has been made towards solving the problem of prevention. There are certainly many causes, and a genetic abnormality is one. An interesting piece of research has therefore been carried out in collaboration with John Burn, Professor of Medical Genetics, on the risks of malformations appearing in the offspring of those already so afflicted.

(e) Disease of the Lungs. In addition to the effect, noted above, of heart disease damaging the lungs, the latter may do the opposite. The combination of Echo and Doppler has made it possible both to diagnose and to assess the severity of 'Hyaline Membrane Disease', a serious lung malady of babies, and so assist in its management.

3. Hypertension. Although high blood pressure is a malady, whose effects on the heart are very important, and whose treatment is very often in the hands of the cardiologist, in Newcastle research upon it has in greatest part been conducted by Robert Wilkinson, Professor of Renal Medicine and his staff in the Department of Nephrology. That research falls into the following categories:

(a) In early years, the late 1970s and 1980s, the significance of renin, a substance derived from the kidney, was investigated in relation to hypertension and disease of the kidneys, including renal artery stenosis. The effects of treatment, both surgical and medical, have been evaluated. More recently a collaborative study with workers in Glasgow has identified what factors determine the outcome, when patients have both kidney disease and high blood pressure.

(b) Investigations have been carried out into the mechanism whereby diabetic patients are prone to develop hypertension and into what are the most appropriate methods of treatment.

(c) 'Sodium/lithium countertransport'. By using a method involving the electrolyte transport properties of red blood cell membranes, they have been able to identify individuals, who, for genetic reasons, are likely to develop high blood pressure, high levels of lipids in their blood and a tendency to premature atherosclerosis.

Altogether in Newcastle, research into the maladies of the human heart has never been so active as it is today. Professor Sir William Hume would have been most impressed.

Notes

1. Mackenzie, J., (a) *The Study of the Pulse, Arterial, Venous, and Hepatic, and of the Movements of the Heart.* McMillan Co. of New York and London 1902.
   (b) The Ink Polygraph. *Br. Med. J.* 1908; 1: 1411.
2. Hume, W. E., (a) A case in which high speed of the auricles did not produce tachycardia. *Quart. J. Med.* 1913; 6: 235–41.
   (b) A Polygraphic Study of 4 Cases of Diphtheria with a Pathological Study of 3 cases. *Heart* 1913–14; 5: 25–44.
3. Szekely, P., Snaith, L., The heart in toxaemia of pregnancy. *Br. Heart J.* 1947; 9: 128–36.
4. Szekely, P., Snaith, L., The place of cardiac surgery in the management of the pregnant woman with heart disease. *J. Obst. Gynaec.* 1963; 70: 69–73.
5. Szekely, P., Snaith, L., *Heart disease and pregnancy.* Edinburgh: Churchill Livingston, 1974.
6. Swan, W. G. A. Acute non-specific pericarditis. *Br. Heart J.* 1960; 22: 651–9.
7. Swan, W. G. A., Dewar, H. A. The heart in haemochromatosis. *Br. Heart J.* 1952; 14: 117–24.
8. Court, S. D. M. *The medical care of children.* London: Oxford Univ. Press, 1963.
9. Szekely, P., Bethune, M. B. Rheumatic fever and rheumatic heart disease – natural history and preventive aspects. *Public Hlth.* 1964; 78: 78–84.
10. Hill, I. G. W., Dewar, H. A. Effort Syndrome. *Lancet* 1945; 2: 161–4.
11. Dewar, H. A., Horler, A. R., Cassells-Smith, A. J. Fibrinolytic treatment of coronary thrombosis – a pilot study. *Brit. Med. J.* 1961; 2: 671–5.
12. Dewar, H. A., Stephenson, P., Horler, A. R., Cassells-Smith, A. J., Ellis, P. A. Fibrinolytic Therapy of Coronary Thrombosis. Controlled Trial of 75 Cases. *Br. Med. J.*, 1, 915–20.
13. Menon, I. S., Dewar, H. A. Increased fibrinolytic activity in venous blood of hemiplegic limbs. *Br. Med. J.* 1967; 2: 613–5.
14. Amery, A., Roeber, G., Vermeulen, H. J., Verstraete, M. Single-blind randomised multicentre trial comparing heparin and streptokinase treatment in recent myocardial infarction. *Acta med. Scand.* 1969; Supp 505: 5–37.

15. Hall, R. J. C., Dewar, H. A. Safety of coronary arterial prostacyclin infusion (letter). *Lancet* 1981; 1: 949.

16. Saran, R. K., Been, M., Furniss, S. S., Hawkins, T., Reid, D. S. Reduction in ST Segment elevation after thrombolysis predicts either coronary reperfusion or preservation of left ventricle function. *Br. Heart J.* 1990; 64(2): 113–7.

17. Julian, D. G., Prescott, R. J., Jackson, F. J., Szekely, P. Controlled trial of sotalol for one year after myocardial infarction. *Lancet* 1982, 1, 1143–7.

18. Julian, D. G. Should ACE inhibitors be administered to all patients after acute myocardial infarction? A (cautious) negative response [Review]. *Europ. Heart J.* 1995; Suppl. E: 44–5.

CHAPTER 6

CARDIAC SURGERY AND THE REGIONAL CARDIOTHORACIC SURGICAL UNITS

The Regional Cardiothoracic Surgery Service in the North-east began in Newcastle in 1934 with a few courtesy beds at Newcastle General Hospital. Most operations in those days were for pulmonary tuberculosis, bronchiectasis and lung cancer, though post-pneumonic empyema, lung abscess, spontaneous pneumothorax and chest injuries, both civilian and military, were other indications. By the outbreak of the Second World War up to eighty beds were in constant use, with a growing waiting list. The Unit was headed by a Durham graduate, Mr George Mason. He was joined as First Assistant in 1940 by Mr Selwyn Griffin, who had graduated in Liverpool.

Mason was keen to extend the scope of his work to the heart and shortly before the Second World War he met Laurence O'Shaughnessy and under his stimulus did some experimental work on greyhounds and then some cardio-omentopexies. This operation for ischaemic heart disease (already mentioned in the chapter on research) entailed bringing up through the diaphragm the abdominal omentum with its blood supply left intact, and stitching it to the heart in the hope that blood vessels from the omentum would invade the myocardium. He also visited Beck in the U.S.A. who, for the same purpose, was using (of all things!) asbestos to scarify the surface of the heart to encourage adhesions

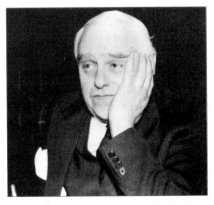

Mr George A. Mason M.B., B.S. (Durham), F.R.C.S. Consultant Cardiothoracic Surgeon, Shotley Bridge General Hospital, 1940–66.

between it and the pericardium. The feasibility of increasing blood flow to the sub-endocardial heart muscle by constricting the coronary sinus was also discussed. None of these measures proved successful and fortunately the war put an end to further research along these lines.

In 1940 the Unit was transferred to Gateshead Emergency Hospital at Stannington as part of a general policy of evacuation and dispersal of patients away from areas of strategic importance. Next year it was transferred to the hutment section of Shotley Bridge Hospital, then known as the Shotley Bridge Emergency Medical Services Hospital, where it occupied five wards comprising 150 beds. The operating theatre, designed for war casualty cases, consisted of one huge room containing four operating tables. This theatre remained in use until late in 1952.

At the end of the war, with the introduction of antibiotics, improved anaesthetic techniques and a reliable blood transfusion service, cardiac surgery became much more promising.

The Unit remained at Shotley Bridge and, to cope with the increasing work load, two additional consultant surgeons were appointed, in 1947 Mr Selwyn Griffin and in 1951, Mr Corbett Barnsley, who had worked under Mr Mason at Newcastle General Hospital. Corbett became a well loved and legendary figure at Shotley Bridge, not least because, despite operating daily on patients with lung cancer, he was an unrepentant chain smoker and was once seen smoking two cigarettes at once! His car could be readily identified by its derelict character and by the pile of cigarette ash overflowing the ash tray and forming a cone on the carpet below it. In 1953 a fourth surgeon, Mr Raymond Dobson, was appointed to share the increasing workload of thoracic cases.

In 1947 Dr Joan Millar was appointed as the first full-time Cardiothoracic Anaesthetist to the Unit. She was immensely loyal to George Mason and would hear nothing against him. She gave unstinting and devoted care to its patients for the next thirty years, and although herself not always in good health, would often sleep in the hospital on nights when particularly sick patients were likely to need her services.

George Mason was a great enthusiast and innovator and in 1950 performed at Shotley Bridge the first mitral valvotomy in the North-east and one of the first in Britain. This was a 'closed' operation, i.e. done without cardiopulmonary bypass, and the mitral valve was dilated by the surgeon's finger inserted through a 'purse-string suture' in the left auricle. He was assisted on that historic occasion by Selwyn Griffin, and Joan Millar gave the anaesthetic. Other closed operations followed – ligation of a patent ductus arteriosus, pulmonary valvotomy and Blalock shunt operations for Tetralogy of Fallot. Several Potts' aorto-pulmonary shunt operations were performed personally by W. J. Potts while a guest of Mason's in Newcastle. Several of those patients are still alive today and two of them have done very well after recent heart-lung and heart transplant operations respectively.

Within a few years the technique of hypothermia was introduced. The anaesthetised patient was placed in a bath of ice and water until the body temperature had fallen to 30°C and this was maintained on the operating table by ice packs around the limbs. This permitted arrest of the circulation by clamping the venae cavae, a technique known as 'inflow occlusion', while surgical correction of the malformation was performed.

By late 1952 the single wartime operating theatre was no longer suitable for the increasing number and complexity of cardiac operations. To enable cardiothoracic surgery to continue, emergency improvements were carried out to the operating theatre and X-ray facilities at Holmside and South Moor Hospital and these opened for use in April 1953. This temporary move enabled work to proceed on a new theatre and X-ray suite on the site of the old theatre at Shotley Bridge. This consisted of two main operating theatres, the larger being spacious enough to accommodate the large number of staff and pieces of equipment it was envisaged would be necessary for cardiac surgical operations of the future, a forecast which was proved accurate when, with the arrival of open-heart surgery, the space was more than adequate. Its facilities included a camera built into the operating lamp and a separate recording and monitoring room. The other somewhat smaller theatre was devoted to thoracic (i.e. non-cardiac) surgery. There was in addition a third smaller theatre catering for bronchoscopies and for treatment of infected cases. In the same suite was a well equipped X-ray room where bronchograms could be performed and a big 'rest room' which was furnished with a large bank of X-ray viewing boxes and doubled as a meeting room in which George Mason conferred with an increasing number of visiting surgeons from this country and overseas. The official opening ceremony of the new theatre suite was performed on 7 May 1955 by Professor Clarence Crafoord, Professor of Thoracic Surgery at Stockholm University.

By 1955 the medical staff of the Unit had grown to five surgeons, five anaesthetists, visiting physicians and cardiologists, (but none specifically appointed to the Unit), and a senior radiologist, Dr Whateley Davidson, who attended twice a week. Former trainees from the Unit were in posts in Australia, Canada, China, Colombia, India, New Zealand and Norway and in Consultant posts in the United Kingdom.

In 1956 a small number of cardiac operations was commenced at Seaham Hall near Sunderland by Selwyn Griffin and other surgeons visiting from Shotley Bridge, the first being ligation of a patent ductus arteriosus. In May 1960 the first open-heart surgical operation at Shotley Bridge using cardiopulmonary bypass was performed by Mason and his team. It was 'patch closure' of an atrial septal defect.

George Mason was a complex character. He had immense drive, gave great attention to detail, and could rely on selfless support from his medical and nursing staff. With a genial personality and a private income, he travelled widely and made many surgical friends whom he invited to Shotley Bridge, where they inspired and charmed his staff. Yet often he did not see his patients before their operations, his ward rounds were infrequent, and he did not personally follow up his patients afterwards. Sadly, the success rate and risk of his operations fell behind many of those elsewhere in the U.K. This led to an increasing number of patients being referred by the cardiologists to other centres outside of the region, particularly to Andrew Logan in Edinburgh. Ironically, Logan had worked at the Royal Victoria Infirmary in Newcastle at the time when Mason was operating at Newcastle General Hospital and had assisted him there.

Partly because of this, and also because of a clash of personalities between Mr Mason and his colleagues, who found him increasingly overbearing and difficult to work with, at the instigation of Adrian Swan in May 1961 a decision was taken by the Regional Health Authority to extend and upgrade the facilities at Seaham Hall to enable open-heart surgery to be performed there. Selwyn Griffin and Raymond Dobson moved to Seaham Hall, accompanied by Dr Henry ('Paddy') Bell, Consultant Anaesthetist. They were joined in 1962 by Dr Joan Errington, who had previously worked in the Unit at Shotley Bridge and later in the Cardiovascular Department at Newcastle General Hospital. As Junior Hospital Medical Officer and later Associate Specialist, she provided the cardiological cover at Seaham, with Charles Henderson providing consultant cover from Newcastle General. In a period of 17 years Griffin, who was a skilful and meticulous surgeon, and his team performed some 2,000 closed mitral valvotomies with an overall mortality rate of 2%. A lesser amount of open-heart surgery, especially that using hypothermia, was also performed, but development of this was constrained by lack of facilities and the limited cardiological cover. He did, however, successfully operate on a series of cases of the 'ostium secundum' type of atrial septal defect with this technique, opening the chest through a lateral incision, which on healing would in a woman become invisible under the left breast. Hypothermia gave the surgeon eight minutes operating time. Selwyn always completed his operations with two minutes to spare. In later years on the, arguably correct, advice of Charles Henderson, no surgery for coronary artery disease was introduced. Although the establishment of this second centre fulfilled at the time its purpose in improving the quality of cardiac surgery in the Northern Region, and stemmed the flow of patients to other centres outside of the region, its throughput of cases could no longer compete with the great increase in the number of operations which were performed at Shotley Bridge following Mason's retirement in 1966.

Until 1965 radiological services to the Cardiothoracic Unit at Shotley Bridge had been provided by visiting radiologists and by the hospital's own general radiologists. In that year Dr William Urquhart was appointed to Newcastle General and Shotley Bridge Hospitals as their first specialist Cardiac Radiologist. He was responsible for a vast improvement and updating of radiological equipment and services in the Cardiothoracic Unit.

In 1966 the appointment of Mr Ary Blesovsky as successor to George Mason at Shotley Bridge General Hospital began a new era in the surgical treatment of cardiological patients in the North-east. Blesovsky ('Bles' to all his friends and colleagues) before his appointment to the Regional Cardiothoracic Surgical Service, had been Senior Registrar, rotating between three major cardiac surgical centres at Barts, National Heart Hospital and the Brompton Hospital. He was thus fully trained in the latest advances in cardiac surgery and

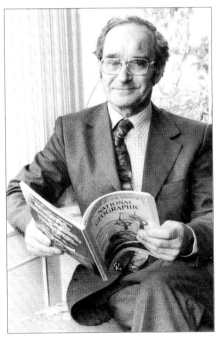

Mr Selwyn G. Griffin M.B., B.S. (Liverpool), F.R.C.S., Consultant Cardio-thoracic Surgeon, Shotley Bridge, Seaham Hall and Freeman Hospitals, 1940–78.

especially in operating with the use of full cardiopulmonary bypass, which by then had largely superseded hypothermia. Bles was enthusiastic, highly skilled and an indefatigable worker. He held very definite views on a number of subjects and would defend them at times quite heatedly. He occasionally summoned his cardiologist colleague into the operating theatre to demonstrate what he regarded as a discrepancy between his finding at operation and those predicted from the clinical and catheter data. He was one of the few surgeons who was also very skilled in the use of a stethoscope and was quite prepared to argue about the precise timing of a mitral 'opening snap', often to the point where a phonocardiogram had to be performed to settle the dispute!

With his arrival at Shotley Bridge, the annual number of open-heart operations increased in the first year from 34 to 178 and their success rate improved so much that Shotley Bridge soon became once again the major cardiac surgical centre in the North-east. In particular, operations for the various forms of congenital heart disease whose correction required more time than had been available with hypothermia were carried out in increasing numbers under full cardiopulmonary bypass. The results were excellent. His previous training under Mr O. S. Tubbs and Sir Russell (later Lord) Brock had given him unique experience of closed mitral valvotomy, using the mechanical valve dilators which had by then made manual dilation of the mitral valve obsolete. He excelled at closed mitral valvotomy and a number of his early patients were still well and free from re-stenosis when he retired some twenty years later. Nevertheless, he was adamant that, provided that the initial closed valvotomy had been performed by a competent operator using mechanical dilation, further attempts at closed valvotomy of a re-stenosed valve were fruitless and the only solution was open valvotomy or, more usually, mitral valve replacement. His results soon justified his views. He meticulously documented by photography the appearance of every valve he removed and demonstrated strikingly that in

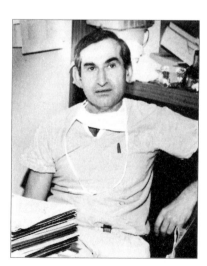

Mr Ary Blesovsky M.B., Ch.B. (Cape Town), F.R.C.S. Consultant Cardiothoracic Surgeon, Shotley Bridge and Freeman Hospital, 1966–89.

the vast majority of cases nothing short of valve replacement would suffice. This was at a time when a number of cardiac surgeons elsewhere were still performing second, third, and even fourth closed valvotomies on often grossly calcified valves and deluding themselves that they had achieved some benefit.

The main constraints on the number of cardiac operations possible at Shotley Bridge were shortage of medical staff and the lack of intensive care beds. Dr Joan Millar continued after George Mason's retirement to provide equally devoted anaesthetic service to his successor and, where necessary, to spend the night after operations in residence at the hospital.

With the greater complexity of cardiac surgery and the need for careful selection of patients, it became obvious that the presence was required of a fully trained cardiologist based at Shotley Bridge. In August 1967 Dr Ronald Gold, who had been a close colleague and fellow Senior Registrar with Bles at the Brompton Hospital in London, was appointed as an additional Consultant Cardiologist to the Regional Cardiology Service, to be based at Shotley Bridge but with outpatient and catheter sessions at Newcastle General Hospital. Gold graduated at Adelaide University, South Australia, in 1952 and came to this country for post-graduate experience in 1957. He decided on a career in cardiology and in order to gain a foothold on the difficult career ladder in that speciality, he forsook his then status of registrar to become house officer to Dr Paul Wood at the Brompton Hospital in London. At Paul Wood's suggestion, he became the first cardiological registrar, then senior registrar at Papworth Hospital, Cambridgeshire, before returning to the Brompton Hospital in May 1962 as senior registrar to Paul Wood. Tragically, Wood, a graduate of Melbourne University and the most brilliant British cardiologist of his generation, died of a myocardial infarction in July 1962. Gold, however, continued as senior registrar there for the next five years.

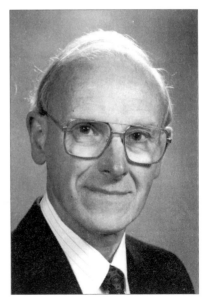

Dr Ronald G. Gold, M.B., B.S. (Adelaide), F.R.C.P. (London and Australia), Consultant Physician, Freeman Hospital, Newcastle upon Tyne, 1987–.

It was there that his intense interest in bedside diagnosis and in particular in cardiac auscultation took root. He also developed his interest in cardiac pacing while at the Brompton, as well as gaining a wealth of experience in cardiac catheterisation of patients both adult and paediatric. His appointment in the Northern Region was achieved proleptically in anticipation of Adrian Swan's retirement four years later.

At the time of Gold's appointment, cardiac catheterisation facilities at Shotley Bridge, although ideally situated next to and in the same sterile environment as the cardiac surgical theatres, were rudimentary. Due to the previous efforts of Bill Urquhart, the radiological equipment in the catheter laboratory was already quite well advanced for its day, with biplane automatic cut film changers and 16 mm ciné cameras for angiography, but equipment for adequate measurement and recording of intracardiac pressures was totally lacking. Nor was there any adequately trained local technician to operate it, the previous sporadic catheterisations having been attended by the Chief Cardiac Technician from Newcastle General Hospital. With a grant from the Regional Health Authority, the necessary new equipment was purchased and a senior and a student technician appointed.

Because of the greatly increased needs for cardiac anaesthesia and development and supervision of the cardiopulmonary bypass equipment, Dr Derek Pearson moved in 1968 from his post as consultant anaesthetist at Newcastle General Hospital, where he had been appointed in 1966, to join Joan Millar as the second full-time cardiac anaesthetist at Shotley Bridge.

Initially, apart from the Consultant Cardiologist, there was only one cardiological registrar to provide the 24-hour cardiological cover necessary for the rapidly increasing activities of the Cardiac Surgery and Cardiology Departments. Early in the nineteen seventies, funding was obtained from the Regional Health Authority for the appointment of a Senior House Officer, on a six-monthly rotation between Dr Robert Mowbray, the Consultant Physician with a cardiological interest at Dryburn Hospital, Durham, and the Cardiology Department at Shotley Bridge. Before that, on the alternate nights when the Cardiological Registrar was off duty, immediate cover was provided by the general medical and cardiac surgical junior staff, but in practice it meant that the Consultant Cardiologist was on call day and night seven days per week. In his absence it was necessary to arrange cover by one of the Consultant Cardiologists at Newcastle General Hospital.

In 1970 the two-bedded recovery area adjacent to the cardiac theatre at Shotley Bridge was replaced by a modern ten-bedded fully monitored cardiac surgical intensive care unit. The monitoring equipment, designed specifically for this by Cardiac Recorders Ltd., was one of the earliest examples of modular plug-in systems incorporating, where necessary, two channels for intravascular pressure measurement.

The catheter laboratory at Shotley Bridge became increasingly busy, especially when surgery for coronary artery disease became routine and demanded pre-operative assessment of all of these patients by coronary angiography. In those days the situation was far from ideal. The catheter laboratory at Shotley Bridge, although, as we have seen, ideally situated for rapid transfer of patients to cardiac surgery, did not have the high definition image intensifiers or good quality ciné equipment available at Newcastle General Hospital. On the other hand, any patient catheterised in Newcastle requiring emergency surgical intervention had to be rushed by ambulance the fifteen miles to Shotley Bridge.

In 1969 transvenous pacemaker implantation was commenced at Shotley Bridge and a full account of this appears in the chapter devoted to Cardiac Pacing.

Because of the increasing work-load in cardiac surgery, in 1974 Mr Michael Holden was appointed as the second Consultant Cardiac Surgeon at Shotley Bridge. He had received his training in Leeds and under Barratt-Boyes in New Zealand and brought with him special expertise in the surgery of congenital heart disease and in homograft and pericardial xenograft valve replacement. He also became an enthusiastic advocate of the two-stage procedure for pacemaker implantation described in more detail in the chapter on Cardiac Pacing, and performed most of the surgical implantations of the 'box' at Shotley Bridge after the 'lead' (the active end) had been put in place in the heart by the cardiologist. Results of this partnership between cardiologist and surgeon proved so successful and uneventful that the procedure continued to be used until 1978, after the opening of Freeman Hospital. By then, pacing leads had become so reliable that the two-stage technique was superseded by a single stage procedure performed solely by a cardiologist.

The end of the 'sixties and early 'seventies brought considerable changes in surgical techniques as well as the rapid growth of coronary artery surgery. By the nineteenth-fifties rheumatic fever in Britain had virtually disappeared. One remembers the excitement caused around 1970 by the admission to Ward 7 of Newcastle General Hospital of a teenager suffering from this now rare illness. However, the legacy from the earlier years of patients subsequently developing rheumatic valvular heart disease continued unabated well into that decade and valve replacement operations remained the commonest cardiac surgical procedures for some years.

Initially open-heart surgery at Shotley Bridge was performed using the Melrose rotating cylinder oxygenator, and in the early days this was not without its problems. Bubble production in the bypass circuit was responsible for an unacceptably high incidence of intra-operative cerebral complications and this topic provided a major research project for Derek Pearson. The advent of the various bubble oxygenators such as the Baxter Bag considerably reduced the frequency of these complications. Nevertheless some problems still remained until membrane oxygenators were introduced. As a result of his research, Pearson became an adviser to the Department of Health on oxygenators and Shotley Bridge and later Freeman Hospital became evaluation centres for them.

Presently the valve prostheses themselves underwent changes of fashion. In the late 'sixties, the silastic ball Starr-Edwards valve with bare metal struts proved very reliable and many of those patients were still alive and well, albeit on anticoagulants, two decades later. Efforts by manufacturers to reduce the risk of embolism from valve prostheses were a mixed blessing. The covering of the struts with cloth, which soon frayed, produced haemolysis, often severe. Changing the silastic ball for one of metal fared similarly and also produced a new physical sign – opening and closing sounds from the valve clearly audible without a stethoscope. Indeed one patient, sitting next to a stranger in a bus, remarked 'So you have one too'! A disc valve designed by Beall, although quiet and with a small risk of embolism, proved a universal failure. Due to wear of the disc against the struts of the supporting cage, regurgitation (leaking) occurred or, worse still, obstruction due to jamming of the disc. Homografts enjoyed temporary popularity because patients with them did not need anticoagulants, but these valves wore out quite quickly and the surgical work-load was further increased by the need for second valve replacements. Pericardial and porcine xenograft valves fared somewhat better, but after about ten years these too often required replacing. As the late effects of rheumatic infections gradually disappeared, aortic valve disease became more common than new cases of mitral valve disease, for many of these were due to the stenosis and calcification of congenital bicuspid valves, and presented in middle age.

From 1973 onwards, increasing attention was directed to the planning of the new Freeman Hospital and the unification of the cardiac services of the region. Staff of the Shotley Bridge Cardiothoracic Unit were heavily involved in this and the Cardiac Surgical Intensive Care Unit was used as a site for the evaluation and testing of the patient monitoring equipment for the new hospital.

The move of the entire Cardiothoracic Unit from Shotley Bridge was a mammoth undertaking but went remarkably smoothly and, although all but emergency heart operations had to be suspended for several weeks beforehand, this presented few problems in the management of patients. A number of the nursing staff and technicians, particularly those working in the cardiothoracic theatres, elected to move to Freeman Hospital with the Unit, while others were transferred to other duties at Shotley Bridge Hospital.

The admission of the first patients to the new cardiac and thoracic surgical wards at Freeman Hospital took place on 12 October 1977, bringing to an end a partnership between Shotley Bridge Hospital and the Regional Cardiothoracic Surgical Unit which had existed for 36 years.

Selwyn Griffin retired in May 1978 on his 65th birthday, shortly after the closure of his department at Seaham Hall. Although, so near his retirement, he had elected not to move to Freeman Hospital, his enthusiasm for surgery was not diminished and during the next two years he helped Hewan Dewar with some published research work on the possibility of treating certain types of bacterial endocarditis with a combination of antibiotics and fibrinolytic agents. Sadly, in March 1992 he suffered a dissection of the aorta while leaving a Rugby match at Murrayfield and died very soon after. He will be remembered not only for his contributions to cardiac surgery in the Region but also for his always courteous and enthusiastic personality.

Raymond Dobson, David Girling and Paddy Bell elected to move into Freeman Hospital but Bell moved on after only a few months and Dobson retired in 1980. Joan Errington also moved from Seaham Hall and provided many years of valuable service at Freeman Hospital as Associate Specialist at various outpatient clinics and in particular, the pacemaker clinics, before retiring in 1992. With the amalgamation of the two surgical centres under the one roof, one might have expected a 'them and us' situation to have arisen. This was not at all the case and members of the two previously rival organisations worked together in excellent harmony as cardiac surgery embarked on a new and exciting era.

The vacancy created by Selwyn Griffin's retirement was filled in 1978 by the appointment of Mr Arthur Hedley Brown. Hedley hailed originally from Newcastle but had in the interim worked in New Zealand and at St Thomas's Hospital, London. He had a particular interest in coronary artery surgery and also carried out research in the animal laboratory at the University. He invented a new style of chest wall retractor, which facilitated the surgical approach for dissecting out the internal mammary arteries. He was also noted for a prodigious appetite, particularly at the Cardiac Club dinners, and for a violent antipathy to added dietary salt. He also regarded anyone who was not extremely lean as being over-weight, and many and loud were the protestations from such patients at being put on the Marriott diet, which made hospital food even less tasty. He jogged regularly from his home to Freeman Hospital and while undoubtedly very physically fit, his appearance when climbing up the incline in Castle Farms Road from Jesmond Dene gave no indication of this. Indeed, when passing him in one's car it was difficult to decide whether to offer him a lift or to run him over to put him out of his apparent misery! When the second cardiac surgical centre was established at South Cleveland Hospital in 1994, Hedley volunteered to move there to help initiate cardiac surgery.

With the expansion of cardiac surgery following the opening of Freeman Hospital, a succession of further anaesthetic appointments were made over the next few years. The first of these was Dr David Heaviside, who became responsible for the running of the resuscitation services throughout the hospital and for the training of junior medical and nursing staff in cardiopulmonary resuscitation.

In 1979 Mr Colin Hilton, who had also received his early surgical training in Newcastle, but who in the interim had worked at Papworth and Harefield Hospitals, was appointed as an additional Consultant Cardiothoracic Surgeon. This was made possible by the retirement of Mr Raymond Hoffmann, a thoracic surgeon at Poole Hospital, which was then closing.

Ray Dobson retired in 1980 and was replaced by Mr Graham Morritt, who, although appointed primarily as a Thoracic Surgeon, also per-formed a considerable amount of cardiac surgery. Corbett Barnsley retired in 1982 and tragically died a few weeks later, not, as many and perhaps he himself had expected, of lung cancer, but of a catastrophic stroke. He was not immediately replaced. Instead, agreement was reached with the University that the NHS funding of this post would be placed at the disposal of the University for the creation of an academic post in Cardiothoracic Surgery. This was eventually achieved, and Mr Chris McGregor was appointed as Senior Lecturer in 1984. It was clear from the outset that McGregor was determined to make Freeman Hospital the third U.K. centre for Cardiac Transplantation and it therefore came as no surprise when, with private funding from the U.S.A., he embarked upon a programme of heart transplants in 1985 without waiting for a decision from the Department of Health, to whom formal application for this had been made. Eventually, confronted with a fait accompli, the Department of Health ratified Freeman Hospital as the third transplant centre. Having achieved his goal, McGregor then left to take up a post at the Mayo Clinic in the U.S.A.

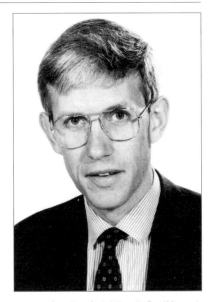

Mr. John Dark M.B., B.S. (Newc.), F.R.C.S. (Eng. and Ed.), Cardio-thoracic Surgeon and Director of Cardio-pulmonary Transplants, Freeman Hospital, Newcastle upon Tyne, 1987–.

He was replaced in 1987 by Mr John Dark, a Newcastle graduate, who continued as Director of the Cardiac Transplantation Unit and Consultant Cardiothoracic Surgeon. Under his guidance the transplant programme thrived and its needs soon outstripped the facilities available. To provide for the strict isolation of transplant patients in the early post-operative period, the ten-bedded cardiac surgical Intensive Care Unit had been modified, with the loss of two beds. In 1990 a five-bed extension to the unit was opened by the then Chairman of the Northern Regional Health Authority, Professor Sir Bernard Tomlinson. The foundation stone of the building extension, designed to accommodate the extended Intensive Care Unit and below it a new suite of offices and laboratories for the Transplant Department, had been laid in 1989 by Princess Diana. Her visit produced great excitement among the patients whom she visited that day. One very elderly lady who had just received a pacemaker, and with whom the Princess had shaken hands, vowed that she would never again wash that hand!

The larger numbers of patients requiring frequent outpatient follow-up necessitated the transfer of the Transplant Outpatient clinics to separate accommodation in a new extension of the Cardiothoracic Unit on the ground floor under the extension to the Intensive Care Unit. The cardiac biopsies which were such an integral part of the monitoring of transplant patients in order to detect early signs of rejection of the donor organ, were performed in Theatre 5 of the Cardiothoracic Theatre Suite. This had originally been designed with a reversible air-flow system to provide for treatment of 'dirty' cases and for bronchography and bronchoscopy cases, but was increasingly used for pacemaker implantation. The result was considerable difficulty in accommodating the conflicting needs of the different specialities, a problem further aggravated by the growth of electrophysiological investigations beyond what could be accommodated in the cardiac catheterisation laboratories, and the transfer of some of these to Theatre 5. The problem was eventually resolved in 1993 when transplant biopsies were moved to new accommodation within the Transplant Department on the ground floor of the Cardiothoracic Department.

In 1988 Mr Raj Behl, who at the time was a Senior Registrar on the Cardiothoracic Surgical Unit, became a Consultant on the unit. It was intended that he should take over much of the paediatric cardiac surgery, but in the event he also carried out an increasing amount of adult cardiac surgery so that the paediatric cardiac surgical needs were still not being met. He resigned in 1992 to work in the Middle East.

In 1989 Ary Blesovsky took early retirement. Unfortunately, in his early days as a keen Rugby football player in South Africa, he had sustained injuries to his knees, which developed into osteo-arthritis. This made standing still at the operating table more and more painful, although it was less of a limitation when he was walking about. He retired to the Isle of Arran. He was succeeded by Mr Leslie Hamilton, who came from Northern Ireland and had had extensive experience as a paediatric cardiac surgeon. His appointment was designed to meet the need for a specialist paediatric cardiac surgeon, a role which he fulfilled admirably, as well as taking part in the on-call rota for adult surgery. In 1990 Derek Pearson took early retirement and went to live in the Lake District.

By the late 1980s coronary artery surgery had come to dominate the cardiac surgical repertoire and the resultant increase in the open-heart surgery load necessitated expansion from the two existing cardiac surgical operating theatres into a third theatre, previously used mainly for thoracic surgical operations. Even this was eventually to prove inadequate, and discussions were commenced regarding the feasibility of a second cardiothoracic surgical centre in the south of the Region. After lengthy deliberation and bids from Hartlepool, North Tees and South

Cleveland Hospitals, it was decided to establish a new cardiac surgical centre at South Cleveland and to expand the Cardiology Department already there. The new unit opened in 1994 and, as already mentioned, Hedley Brown elected to move there to initiate the surgical service. He was followed there in 1995 by Graham Morritt. This decentralisation of cardiac surgical facilities represented a major change in policy, which previously had decreed that the then fragmented cardiac surgical facilities of the region should be centred on Freeman Hospital in Newcastle, and which had resulted in the closure of the units at Shotley Bridge and Seaham Hall. It will fall to the lot of future writers of the history of cardiac surgery in the region to assess the full impact of this development on the Regional Cardiothoracic Service as a whole, and this point would seem an appropriate place to draw this present chronicle of its history to a close.

CHAPTER 7

THE NEWCASTLE CARDIAC CLUB AND THE NORTHERN REGIONAL CARDIOLOGY GROUP

PART I BY H. A. DEWAR.
THE NEWCASTLE CLUB, 1950–1994

With the introduction in 1948 of the National Health Service, came an enormous expansion of the numbers of hospital consultants. Neither the Association of Physicians of Great Britain and Ireland (founded by Sir William Osler in 1907) nor the British Cardiac Society (successor to the British Cardiac Club, whose foundation Hume had initiated in 1922) were likely to be able to offer membership to so many potential candidates. Accordingly Hume, appreciative of the pleasure and the benefit he had himself derived from both, decided to found their equivalents in the Northern Region.

On 11 December 1949 he invited three physicians, two surgeons and one radiologist to meet at his house to form the Newcastle Cardiac Club. They were Corbett Barnsley (Thoracic Surgeon, Shotley Bridge), Whately Davidson (Radiologist, Royal Victoria Infirmary, Newcastle), Hewan Dewar (Physician, R.V.I.), George Mason (Thoracic Surgeon, Shotley Bridge), Robert Mowbray (Physician, Dryburn Hospital, Durham), Adrian Swan (Physician, Newcastle General Hospital) and Paul Szekely (Physician, N.G.H.). With Hume himself, members would number eight. But Hume early suggested that a number of general physicians in the Region with a special interest in heart disease should also be members, so to Mowbray were added Conrad Bremer (Sunderland), Alun Williams (Middlesbrough) and Blair Edmunds (Darlington). They would meet four times a year on a Sunday evening at each others' houses in rotation. The usual pattern would be a paper on a pre-selected topic by one of the members or by a guest speaker, followed by discussion of that paper, then supper (provided by the host) and finally a discussion of interesting cases which members had encountered and of which they would bring details, including X-rays, ECG's or slides of them. This initial composition of the Club owed to Hume three important features, namely that membership would be open to Regional as well as to Teaching Hospital physicians, that radiologists had much to contribute, and that wives could be relied upon to produce good meals, provided it was only for infrequently repeated special occasions. As to the last of these, he demonstrated his own confidence three years later when as President of the British Cardiac Society at its meeting in Newcastle in 1953 he invited all 15 members of its Council to dinner at his house and only told his wife afterwards. Being French and very devoted, she provided a memorable meal. No subscription to the Club was levied until the 113th meeting in 1986, when the numbers attending reached 17 and an annual sum of £2 each was thought appropriate to finance a small gesture of appreciation to the hostesses.

The first proper meeting of the Club took place, again at Hume's house, at 6.00 p.m., on 29 January 1950 and at this meeting it was decided to invite Selwyn Griffin, Thoracic Surgeon, Shotley Bridge General Hospital, also to become a member. Swan introduced the subject of the operative treatment of hypertension and after supper the following cases were discussed: arsenical poisoning with gangrene of the feet, congenital heart defect, and trauma of the heart.

Meetings continued to be held on Sundays until 24 January 1953, which was a Saturday, after which they took place sometimes on Saturday and sometimes on Sunday, until 27 April 1957, when it was decided that Saturday would always be the day. This decision seems to have coincided with a reduction of frequency to 3 meetings a year. On 6 April 1952 it was decided to restrict membership to 12 with up to three extra (guest) members elected for a year at a time. For the first 10 years actual attendance at meetings varied between 5 and 11. Professor Hume himself, owing to severe osteoarthritis of hip, was only occasionally able to attend unless the meeting was in his own house, and his last attendance was on 15 February 1958. Two years later he died aged 81.

The criteria of membership were special interest in heart disease and consultant status or nearly so (Senior Registrars and Senior Lecturers were sometimes admitted as guests, i.e. temporary members). Resignation on retirement had to be insisted upon – except of course for Hume, who was 70 years old when he founded the Club. One other exception was also a founder member, Whately Davidson, the radiologist, who tendered his resignation at 65, was given honorary membership, and continued both to work for the NHS and to attend meetings of the Club until he suddenly died at 80![1] The Club continued to expand and a full list of members with specialities and affiliations is attached as an appendix. From earliest days it was appreciated how much benefit would come from inviting non-members, often from other disciplines and from both the Northern and other Regions, to be guests at a particular meeting where they would introduce a topic on which they were experts or in which they had special experience. Ian Rannie, R.V.I. pathologist, was the first and discussed 'Isolated Myocarditis'. Others followed initially at a rate of one or two a year, but later much more often.

Subjects Discussed

A complete list of topics discussed at the 125 meetings of the Club would make tedious reading, but a summary of them is interesting and is available only because of the excellent minutes kept by the secretaries between 1950 and 1990. A few are quite perennial. The surgical treatment of ischaemic heart disease was discussed at the very first meeting in 1950 and again at the Club's 123rd in 1990. Szekely gave a talk on Heart Disease and Pregnancy at the third meeting in 1950 and Steve Robson described the Haemodynamic Changes in Pregnancy at the 116th in 1987. Dr Michael Oliver (with Professor Duguid) came as an expert guest in 1959 to talk on Diet and Coronary Atheroma and in 1996 the subject is just as debatable. Some topics have almost disappeared – syphilitic damage to the aorta, acute rheumatism, tuberculous pericarditis. Some remain but are much better managed – hypertension, coronary thrombosis and angina, and congenital defects of the heart. A few new ones have appeared – immunological and viral myocarditis, fibrinolysis, and heart transplants. Hume would have been surprised to know that the Club had welcomed a solicitor[2] to talk about 'Innovations and the Law' and that a General Manager of a Health Authority[3] had been invited to speculate on 'What happens in the next five years?' He would have been delighted to learn that the Club had strayed from more serious matters to enjoy Dr Alistair Brewis[4] on 'On and around about the Town Moor'. He would have been even more pleased that it had invited a medical student[5] to describe his research into 'The metabolic effects of hypothermia in children'.

Two other features of these meetings were of particular value. One was the opportunity, first taken by Szekely in 1956, for a member or members who had been to an international cardiological congress to give an account of it to the other members of the Club. The other was the beginning of what would later be called Medical Audit, i.e. the presentation by a member or visitor of some new method of investigation or more especially of treatment for others to appraise.

One problem, ultimately insoluble, was the quite inevitable limitation on numbers of members, especially as appointments of cardiologists expanded. Presentation of a topic or of a case before several colleagues of equal status in the relaxed, friendly and comfortable atmosphere of a private house promotes a candid and detailed discussion of a quality which cannot be matched in the formal setting of a lecture theatre. Also in those earlier days it was possible, as we have seen, to include in the membership a small number of consultants from Regional Hospitals (Dryburn, Sunderland, Darlington and Middlesbrough) with much benefit to everybody. But the difficulty of finding a room large enough and of providing a meal for more than 15 people was too formidable. By the 58th meeting, 17 years after its formation, the limit set by the Club of 12 full-time and three guest members had meant that several consultants with exclusive interests in cardiology were being denied membership altogether or were categorised as temporary guest members year after year until death or retirement created a vacancy. So guest membership was abolished and the number of ordinary members was increased to 16. But the problem persisted and worsened. In 1981 Terry, who was both a member and a Regional physician (Dryburn), partially solved it by founding the Northern Regional Cardiology Group, of which he gives a separate account elsewhere. Nevertheless, by the late 1980s membership had leapt to 29 and actual attendances were running at 17. In 1990 Colin Hilton asked to be relieved of the secretarial duty and Keith Evemy was appointed in his place, but no further meetings were arranged.

In 1994 Dewar, the only surviving founding member, hearing that the Club was dormant if not moribund, wrote to Campbell offering to host a 125th and possibly final meeting, both as a celebration of his recent 80th birthday and as a stimulus to reaching a decision on the Club's future. The meeting took place at Dewar's home in Wylam on 7 July. Professor Keith Fox of Edinburgh gave a talk on 'Fibrinolysis and the Heart' and after a buffet meal, Dewar recounted a short history of the Club. After this meeting, at Campbell's request, Evemy circulated to all members a letter and questionnaire (a rather similar one had been circulated in 1986, also with an equivocal result.) Of the 14 replies received, not all of them complete, and comprising about half of the total circulated, most indicated that they wished the Club to continue in a modified form and that the meetings should not be in members' houses, but in a hotel/restaurant. Campbell then devised a new format for them, but when this was circulated only three replies were received, two favourable one against. It was concluded that members' enthusiasm was so small that the Club should terminate.

Notes

1. Dr Samuel Whateley Davidson was a most remarkable and delightful man. M.R.C.P. by examination, he intended to become a consultant physician, but was persuaded by Hume to become a radiologist and had a most distinguished career. Immensely energetic, he used to invite his registrar to meet him at his home at 5.00 a.m. for breakfast, then drive the 15 miles to Shotley Bridge Hospital where he would report on yesterday's X-rays and return ready for work at the R.V.I. in Newcastle by 9.00 a.m. Not believing that X-ray facilities should be provided except in its designated department, he opposed Dewar's request for a screening unit in the Dept. of Cardiology. Chairman of the Medical Advisory Committee which met to consider the matter, he found the Committee equally divided and gave his casting vote, by uncharacteristic error from his point of view, the wrong way! – but was too generous to reverse the decision. On 30 August 1977 at the age of 80 he drove to the Queen Elizabeth Hospital in Gateshead, where he was doing a locum, wrote his reports as usual between 6.30 and 9.00 a.m., returned home and died of a cerebral haemorrhage before the reports had reached the wards.

   Many might envy this as an elegant way of saying goodbye.
2. Arthur Taylor M.A., Chairman of Newcastle Health Authority, on 2 July 1983.
3. Charles Marshall, Esq. District General Manager of Newcastle Health Authority, on 9 June 1990.
4. Dr R. A. L. Brewis M.D. F.R.C.P., Consultant Physician, Royal Victoria Infirmary, on 22 October 1983.
5. Eugene M. G. Milne, now M.Sc., M.B. B.S., M.R.C.P., M.F.P.H.M. R.C.P., on 6 November 1983.

PART II BY G. TERRY. NORTHERN
REGIONAL CARDIOLOGY GROUP 1981–1994

On my appointment as Consultant Physician/Cardiologist at Dryburn Hospital in 1979, I was invited to become a member of the Newcastle Cardiac Club. I found this to be an excellent way of hearing about new developments in my speciality as well as enjoying informal meetings with other cardiological colleagues, in the pleasant surroundings of members' homes.

At that time, major changes were occurring in Cardiology in the Northern Region. With the opening of Freeman Hospital there was a large expansion in the number of specialists in the field of Cardiology, Cardiothoracic Surgery and allied disciplines. Also at that time many district general hospitals in the Region were appointing new physicians with special training in Cardiovascular Medicine.

The Newcastle Cardiac Club, which was founded in 1950, could clearly not embrace this large number of extra cardiological colleagues if it remained in its original format, as the size of members' homes could not accommodate the numbers of potential members it would involve. Realising the value of such meetings for continuing education and informal discussion amongst colleagues, in 1980 I contacted one physician in each district of the Northern Region to see if there was an interest in forming a group which would meet on regular occasions to discuss cardiological matters.

I contacted the consultant in each district who was either training in cardiology or who had shown the most interest in the speciality whilst being a 'general physician'. My idea was to bring together D.G.H. physicians who shared an interest in cardiology and invite colleagues from the Regional Cardiothoracic Centre at Freeman Hospital as speakers to keep us up to date with advances in our speciality.

The response was overwhelmingly in favour of forming such a group and our inaugural meeting took place in Durham on 12 June 1981, our guest speaker being Prof. Desmond Julian.

The inaugural members of the group are shown in Table 1.

Subsequent meetings were held in various districts of the Region and the local member hosted the meeting. Our three members in Cumbria attended many meetings which were on the east side of the Pennines. Once each year we held a meeting in the Lake District, which they hosted. This meeting took place over a weekend in autumn and, in addition to education and informal discussion, encompassed a certain degree of fell-walking.

Over the years, not only did we utilise our colleagues at Freeman Hospital as speakers, but we also arranged speakers from other Regions to come and share their expertise with us.

One of our most memorable meetings occurred in Durham in 1984. I heard on the grapevine that Sir Brian Barratt-Boyes was visiting New-castle and wrote to him, inviting him to speak to the group. To my delight he readily agreed to come and talk about his vast experience in valve replacement surgery. On this occasion we invited members of the New-castle Cardiac Club and other members of staff from Freeman Hospital. A very enjoyable evening ensued.

The activities of the group were always strongly supported by our first speaker, Desmond Julian, and it was with a mixture of joy and sadness that he spoke to us again in 1986 as he left Newcastle to take up his appointment as Medical Director of the British Heart Foundation. Un-fortunately for him he still could not escape from us, for in 1991 we invited him back to talk to us on the work of the B.H.F.!

A list of the meetings of the Group is shown in Table 2.

Unfortunately, by the early 1990s, meetings of the group became less frequent and less well attended. The reason for this is not entirely clear but this fall-off coincided almost exactly with the time that the Royal Colleges were asking consultants to document their CME activities for the purposes of continuing accreditation!

I can only hope that the group can be re-established as we are now moving into another era in Cardiology in the Northern Region. A second Regional Centre has now been established in South Cleveland and now every D.G.H. in the 'old' Northern Region has a trained cardiovascular physician in post and many now have two!

INAUGURAL MEMBERS – NRCG

L. G. BRYSON	SOUTH SHIELDS
E. A. CAMERON	ASHINGTON
A. DAVIES	SOUTH CLEVELAND
D. M. DAVIES	SHOTLEY BRIDGE
G. H. EVANS	TYNEMOUTH
K. EVEMY	NEWCASTLE
A. L. GIBSON	GATESHEAD
J. HAMPSON	DARLINGTON

G. ISMAY	BISHOP AUCKLAND
F. LOCAL	WHITEHAVEN
B. MITTRA	SUNDERLAND
R. H. ROBSON	CARLISLE
G. B. RYDER	HEXHAM
R. H. SMITH	NORTH TEES
C. A. SYKES	BARROW in FURNESS
G. TERRY	DURHAM
R. B. WHITE	HARTLEPOOL

CHAPTER 8

TEACHING

One of the charms of cardiology is that so much useful information can be obtained by using three of the five senses – looking, feeling and listening, and the pleasure of teaching medical students lies in training them to use them. Over the years, the settings for instruction have changed but the principles remain the same.

Until the end of the Second World War, the outpatient setting was of general physicians on the staff of the Royal Victoria Infirmary seeing and teaching on all manner of illnesses, some of them cardiological. They would include maladies such as rheumatic valvular disease, atherosclerosis with and without high blood pressure, and syphilis. There might also be examples of congenital malformations, but not much instruction was given about them. There was no satisfactory treatment and to students the differential diagnosis appeared a miracle of consultant expertise. Many children were seen at the Fleming Memorial Hospital for Sick Children, but it was not regarded as a proper part of the teaching group, so that not all students attended there. Hume used only to see a few cases of heart disease in the 'dayroom', attached to his male ward, preparatory to starting his twice-weekly ward round. Only Assistant Physicians did whole morning outpatient clinics, and follow-up sessions would often be allocated to the registrar or house physician. But the assistant physicians did teach, and several such as Dr (later Professor) Fred Nattrass did so brilliantly.

In the wards opportunities for learning about heart disease were in some ways rather better. Many cases were admitted for investigation and many more for treatment, especially of heart failure. X-ray and three-lead electrocardiograms were the standard methods of investigation, so that students had good opportunities for familiarising themselves with the pictures, though only the former method was accompanied by a report. The greatest benefit came from the length of stay of the patients. Three weeks was fairly common. The greatest obstacle to instruction was the absence of instructors! Only Dr Horsley Drummond attended every day, and the single medical registrar had many other duties. The assistant physicians (there were four of them), each with only four beds in the men's ward and two in the women's, hesitated to intrude on their 'chiefs' province. The Newcastle General Hospital, with much general medicine, including heart disease, and Walkergate Hospital, where the cases of diphtheritic myocarditis were cared for, were not 'teaching institutions'. The social consequences of heart ailments were hardly taught at all.

The third setting for students was the lecture theatre. Who gave the lectures there was a matter of seniority. If the person who undertook the task was especially gifted, as Hume was, then the result was excellent. But if, as happened in some other disciplines, the teacher allocated the duty because of seniority and supposed interest was not, the effect could be disastrous. Indeed Henry Miller (later Vice-Chancellor of the University) in his student days hired a Salvation Army Band to play outside the lecture theatre in the Northumberland Road Medical School to drown the lecturer's uninformative drone. 'Clinical lectures', i.e. lectures with a patient present, were also given each week in the R.V.I. and sometimes would concern a patient with a heart condition. Since the site was the Consultants Dining Room, where there was only a six-inch raised platform and no tiering of the seats, visibility was very poor. It was only during the 1939–45 war years that Dr C. N. Armstrong, then Clinical Sub-dean, raised the money to begin building and furnishing the new lecture theatre, now so fittingly named after him. Medical students were in fact exceptionally fortunate in their lecturer when they were studying heart disease.

After the Second World War, the introduction of the National Health Service in 1947, the ever widening use of antibiotics and developments in techniques of investigation and treatment of heart disease had a huge impact on teaching, mostly for the better. In any case the need was much greater because the number of medical students gradually tripled.

Firstly the settings increased. As already noted, the Regional Cardiovascular Unit was set up in the Newcastle General Hospital, with old but up-dated premises, and in due course a specially designed coronary care unit was added. There were therefore ample facilities for both in-patient and out-patient instruction, and the students took full advantage of them. At the R.V.I. the Cardiac Department developed from the single room in the basement to 'custom-built' premises where E.C.G.s, now of 12 leads, were taken and a report furnished upon them. An X-ray screening apparatus was installed. Most importantly, there was room for as many out-patient clinics, for either new or return cases, as the consultant and his junior staff could manage. In the cubicles students had reasonable time to examine the patients. Gordon Flanagan of the Dept. of Medical

Physics invented and installed there a singular teaching device. It involved primarily a gramophone disc with black smears on it which reproduced heart sounds and murmurs, any of which could be faded in and out by the turning of a knob. It imitated most accurately, and at a tenth of the cost, the properties of a £2,000 instrument, at that time only available from the U.S.A. Dewar and his staff, however, also retained facilities in the main outpatient department of the Hospital for both himself and his staff.

Secondly there was a substantial increase in the number and quality of both consultants and juniors available for the student. At the N.G.H., Hume himself had an appointment for a few years after retiring from the R.V.I., but the main body of teaching was done by Adrian Swan, Paul Szekely, Fred Jackson and Charles Henderson, with Marion Bethune (later Farmer) instructing on children. They were all very good. At the R.V.I. Dewar continued as the only predominantly cardiac physician, but his consultant colleagues also had some cases of heart disease under their care and took pleasure in teaching on them. Dewar also had several junior staff and sometimes also research staff, available for teaching. His wards in the Infirmary also contained an increasing number of heart cases admitted for investigation, as his cardiac work gradually took over from the general medicine which was implied in his original appointment there as a general physician.

Thirdly changes were made in the formal lectures given in all subjects to students. No longer was their success dependent upon the luck of having a single gifted personality. The lectures were 'integrated', i.e. so arranged that for cardiology the anatomy, physiology and pathology of the heart and great vessels were revised, and followed at once by lectures from the cardiologists and cardiac or vascular surgeons most suited to the task. At the end of the series the students were requested to complete a questionnaire (which they were asked not to sign), giving their opinion on any lecturer or on any aspect of the course upon which they wished to comment. In the cardiology course in the 1960s Charles Henderson received the best reports on his lectures, which were well prepared, lucid, practical and given with a strong voice. Marion Bethune's paediatric lectures were also outstanding because, in addition to the same qualities of careful preparation and lucidity, she introduced a very human aspect to them by the personal attendance of a mother and child. The students were on the whole responsible in their criticisms, but also frank. For many years Dewar had the rather delicate task of conveying them privately to the lecturers. With the appointment of Professor Julian in

1975, responsibility for teaching arrangements was of course transferred to him, but neither he nor his successor Campbell took the view that much change was needed. Quite their most valuable innovation was an arrangement for every student to spend two weeks full-time in the cardiovascular department of the Freeman Hospital.

The system of integrated lectures – rather reminiscent of Professor Hume's museum classes of 70 years before – has continued. The students have been most fortunate in the teaching gifts of their two new professors. Ronnie Campbell now receives their accolade as the best lecturer in the cardiology course. They are fortunate too in the paediatric section of their course. After Marion Farmer retired from the duty of giving the lectures on heart disease in children, Stewart Hunter took over for many years. Another paediatric cardiologist, Christopher Wren, is currently in charge of them.

It is obvious that by the 1980s medical students were receiving a very good education in heart disease. Some new developments have helped them. The introduction of echocardiography is one. This technique, consisting, as already described, of the transmission, reflection and recording of very high frequency sound with their display as images on a fluorescent screen is especially valuable for teaching. It demonstrates not only the structures of the heart and how well it fills and empties, but also enables the student to see how the sounds which he hears through a stethoscope link with the movements and shape of the valves of the heart, which he can actually see.

Another is the introduction of paramedics and their training. A medical student, spending a fortnight in a cardiovascular unit, can hardly watch the paramedics' skill in interpreting electrocardiograms and their expertise in techniques of resuscitation without feeling that as an aspiring doctor he ought at least to try to be as good!

A third development which helps the student is the fact that the Chair of Cardiology, generously funded by the British Heart Foundation, is of course deeply committed to research. A university education without awareness of research proceeding would be to leave the student without his curiosity, one of the most valuable parts of the human mind. If it is lost, not only does he lose all desire to become a researcher himself in hospital, but he almost certainly also loses his capacity and desire to carry on research in general practice. No man is properly educated if he has lost the itch to know.

But it would be wrong to conclude that there are no problems. One springs from the intense specialisation which characterises nearly all teaching hospitals today. A student enters a ward or department expecting to encounter there a particular kind of case, instead of having to distinguish it from a number of other maladies, as he would have to do in general practice. Attachment for periods to District General Hospitals goes some way towards remedying this, and in the Northern Region such attachments are widely used. Another problem is the very short time that so many patients now spend in hospital. The student barely has time to interview and examine them, much less to get to know them as individuals, before they are discharged. The solution to the difficulty is not obvious to this historian.

EPILOGUE

With 60 years of acquaintance with cardiology in Newcastle, and having reviewed 90 years of it, one should perhaps attempt some sort of summary, and it is also tempting to point, however vaguely, to the future.

That nothing happened in cardiology in Newcastle before the Second World War, except what Hume himself achieved, is not surprising. The conditions in which he worked with exiguous staff, a small unpaid commitment to the hospital and poorly structured teaching arrangements could not be expected to provoke locally any great advances in knowledge. Research was virtually impossible and the application of advances made elsewhere depended upon the one man. He, to his great credit, by fruitful contacts and his own personality, kept abreast of them and introduced them to the hospital and to the medical community in which he worked.

The introduction in 1947 of the National Health Service effected a total transformation, of which Hume, at 68 years of age, had the vision to see the potential. The establishment of the Regional Cardiovascular Unit at the Newcastle General Hospital, of the Newcastle Cardiac Club and of the Association of Physicians of Region No. 1, together with some valued encouragement of the surgeon, George Mason, at Shotley Bridge, were the products of that vision. All these enterprises prospered, though the Cardiac Club eventually succumbed to the limitation of its own success. This period, regarded by many consultants as the Golden Age of the NHS, lasted more than 40 years. During the later part of it Cardiac Surgery and Academic and Paediatric Cardiology in particular have been responsible for brilliant achievements and show no sign of decline.

From the point of view of Research and of Teaching, the new NHS had an immense impact. The consultant staff, assured of a steady income and helped by adequate numbers of highly intelligent and enthusiastic juniors, were for the first time able to plan and execute research programmes and combine the labours with care of patients and teaching. Two of the most far-sighted and fruitful initiatives taken by the Faculty of Medicine in Newcastle University were the institution of the Med.

Sci. (Bachelor of Medical Science) course for the keenest and most able of the undergraduates, and the decision to expect and enable every postgraduate clinical trainee to spend at least a year in research. The stream of research publications emanating from the N.G.H., the R.V.I. and in due course the Freeman Hospital, a large proportion of them on cardiological subjects, is the result.

The main impact of cardiac research has been upon the action of drugs, the prevention and treatment of coronary atherosclerosis and its complications, the study and management of disturbances of rhythm and the early recognition and treatment of congenital malformations. Valvular heart disease and high blood pressure have been treated to a high standard. The latter, often closely linked with kidney disease, has received from the university recognition of its importance by the award of a personal chair to Robert Wilkinson. The remarkable success of the heart transplant team has also offered opportunities for research and they have not been neglected.

The teaching of undergraduate students has also enormously improved since the start of the NHS. Consultants and their juniors staff have far more time to teach, both in the wards and in the outpatients clinics. Attachments to Regional General Hospitals, as well as some exposure to general practice, have also helped, as have the routine two weeks in the Cardiac Departments of the R.V.I. and Freeman Hospitals. The system of integrated lectures was a much needed reform. As spectators or participants in research, students at least acquire an interest in it and, one hopes, perhaps some envy and aspiration. It is noteworthy that Regional physicians, many with special training and interest in heart disease, now often take part in both the teaching and the research.

In the future lie challenges, no less attractive to the investigator and the practising clinician, far better equipped and arguably better trained in scientific method than was possible in Hume's day. Elucidating the pathological mechanisms which lead to coronary atherosclerosis has already reached an advanced stage. Since the factors appear to be multiple and likely to affect the cherished lifestyle of the public, it appears probable that much of the research of the future will be concerned with how to circumvent the man-made obstacles! Other attractive areas are the part played by viruses, especially enteroviruses (the prevalence of which is particularly high in the North), in the development of cardiomyopathy and perhaps of valve defects, as well as in the various forms of congenital heart disease. Another is the genetic components of high blood pressure, and of ischaemic and congenital heart disease. The most challenging of all is the pathology of old age, i.e. gerontology. Does heart muscle waste in exactly the same way that skeletal muscle does, and can the wasting be prevented? What is the cellular mechanism whereby ageing leads to malfunction of the pace-making and conducting tissues of the heart? The opportunities and potential horrors of gene manipulation are perhaps best left undescribed.

Unfortunately the obstacles to research are increasing. Owing to the activities of the anti-vivisection lobby, animal experiments are becoming more and more difficult and expensive. Human research is inhibited by the use of the emotional word 'guinea-pig', by the intrusiveness of journalists (who see a 'breakthrough', where there is only a dent in the wire), and, especially where new drug treatments are involved, by the public's burgeoning fondness for litigation. It is arguable that much of medical and particularly cardiac research in the future may become feasible only in other countries.

The teaching of medical students has also begun to encounter serious problems. They derive from the short time patients spend in hospital, and from the over-specialised setting in which the patients there are seen, so different from doctors' surgeries and patients' homes. The Deans of Medical Schools have much to think about.

It is hoped that this account of Newcastle Cardiology may help the reader to appreciate what substantial progress has been made over the ninety years it encompasses, and to become acquainted with the many and often colourful personalities who have contributed to that progress.

APPENDIX I

LIST OF COLLABORATORS
WITH DR DEWAR,
NOT MENTIONED IN THE TEXT

Pre-retirement

Clinical	Non-clinical
Agarwal, R. K.	Augusti, K. T.
Benaim, M. E.	Cassels-Smith, A. J.
Brown, R.	Ellis, P. A.
Burke, F. D.	Newell, D. J.
Das, B.	Weightman, D.
Davidson, L .A. G.	Virden, R.
Goodhart, J. M.	
Jenkins, A. R.	
Kendal, R. Y.	
Muscat-Baron, J.	
Owen, S. G.	
Peaston, M. J. T.	
Rowell, N. R.	
Smith, M. J.	
White, R. W. B.	

Post-retirement

Boon, P. J.	Aherne, W. A.
Johnson, C. E.	Barnes, W. S. F.
	Iravani, M. M.
	Jones, M. R.
	Liddell, I.
	Marriner, J.
	Marshall, T.

Oxley, A.
Smith, N. M.
Stappenbeck, R.
Zar, M. A.

STAFF LISTS OF THE CARDIOLOGY UNIT AT FREEMAN HOSPITAL 1986–95

UNIVERSITY OF
NEWCASTLE UPON TYNE
Freeman Hospital

The Chair of Cardiology

Held by
Professor R. W. F. Campbell
BSc MB ChB FRCP (Ed/Lond)
1986

STAFF:

Senior Lecturer:
Dr J. M. McComb

First Assistant:
Dr P. C. Adams (presently on British American Fellowship)
Dr M. Buchalter (locum)

Research Fellows:
Dr J. Bourke
Dr C. Cowan
Dr S Tansuphaswadikul
Dr G. Parry
Dr K Yusoff
Dr Y. T. Tai
Dr R. Karnik

Senior Technicians:
Mrs L. Harker
Mrs S. Jamieson

Clinical Lecturers: (NHS Consultant Cardiologists)
Dr A. S. Hunter
Dr H. Bain
Dr R. G. Gold
Dr R. Bexton
Dr D. O. Williams
Dr D. S. Reid
Dr R. J. C. Hall

Secretary:
Post Vacant

Associated Staff:
Dr A. Murray (Med.Phys)
Dr C. Griffiths (Med.Phys)
Mr C. Hilton (Consultant Cardiac Surgeon)
Mr C. McGregor (Senior Lecturer in Cardiac Surgery)

GENERAL

Professor D. G. Julian retired from the Chair in 1986. Several events including an international symposium were held in Newcastle to honour him. The national and international reputation of the Newcastle Chair was recognised as a consequence of the energy, enthusiasm and original thinking which he contributed during his 12 year tenure. Professor R. W. F. Campbell took up the appointment at the Chair of Cardiology on 1st May, 1986. Dr J. M. McComb was appointed to the position of Senior Lecturer in the Department. She had previously worked with Dr J. Ruskin, Harvard Medical School, Massachusetts General Hospital, Boston, Massachusetts. Dr P. C. Adams left the Department in February, 1986, to take up his British Heart Foundation British/American Travelling Fellowship at Mount Sinai Hospital in New York with Dr V. Fuster. Dr J. Bourke continues in the Department supported by a British Heart Foundation Research Grant. Dr G. Parry was awarded the Northern Region Research Registrarship. Three Overseas Graduates – Dr K. Yusoff (Malaysia), Dr Y. T. Tai (Hong Kong) and Dr R. Karnik (India) have joined the Department as Research Fellows.

The Department was privileged to have Professor G. Acharya, Professor of Cardiology in Nepal, join the Department for an eight month period under the auspices of the British Council.

RESEARCH

Epicardial repolarisation mapping.

Considerable progress has been made in this research venture. Mr C. Hilton, Dr C. Cowan and Dr C. Griffiths have been those primarily involved in this.

UNIVERSITY OF NEWCASTLE UPON TYNE

Freeman Hospital and
The Catherine Cookson Building
of the New Medical School
1988

The Chair of Cardiology

Held by
Professor R. W. F. Campbell MB ChB, FRCP

STAFF:

Senior Lecturer:
  Dr J. M. McComb

First Assistant:
  Dr J. P. Bourke

Research Fellows:
  Dr S. Furniss
  Dr A. Murtazam
  Dr C. Day
  Dr A. D'Onofrio
  Dr K. Yusoff
  Dr V. Dougenis
  Dr M. Munclinger
  Dr Y. T. Tai

Clinical Lecturers:
  Dr P. C. Adams
  Dr H. H. Bain
  Dr R. S. Bexton
  Dr K. Evemy
  Dr R. G. Gold
  Dr A. S. Hunter
  Dr D. S Reid
  Dr D. O. Williams

Secretarial Staff:
  Miss S. J. Murray
  Mrs D. Naisby (NHS)
  Mrs J. Horsley
  Mrs M. Jopson

Senior Technicians:
  Mrs L. Harker
  Mrs S. Jamieson
  Mr P. Harrison

Associated NHS Staff:
  Dr A. Murray (Medical Physics)
  Mr C. Griffiths (Medical Physics)
  Mr C. J. Hilton (Surgery)

Dr T. Ashcroft (Pathology)
Dr G. Bird (Immunology)
Dr C. Wren (Paediatric Cardiology)
Prof. O. James (Medicine)

UNIVERSITY OF NEWCASTLE UPON TYNE

Freeman Hospital and
The Catherine Cookson Building
of the New Medical School
1989

The Chair of Cardiology

Held by
Professor R. W. F. Campbell, MB, ChB, FRCP

STAFF:

Senior Lecturers:
Dr J. M. McComb (BHF
    funded)
Dr C. Wren (Children's
    Heart Unit funded)

First Assistants:
Dr J. P. Bourke (until 9.88
    BHF funded)
Dr S. S. Furniss (from 9.88
    BHF funded)

Research Fellows:
Dr S. S. Furniss (until 9.88
    – BHF Project Grant funded)
Dr A. Murtazam (Government
    of Malaysia
Dr C. Day (British Digestive
    & BHF funded)
Dr A. D'Onofrio (Italian
    Cardiac Soc. Grant)
Dr K. Nimkhedar (Self-
    supporting)
Dr A. Loaiza (British Council funded)

Clinical Lecturers:
Dr P. C. Adams
Dr H. H. Bain
Dr R. S. Bexton
Dr K. Evemy
Dr R. G. Gold
Dr A. S. Hunter
Dr D. S. Reid
Dr D. O. Williams

Secretarial Staff:
Ms S. J. Murray (BHF
    funded)
Ms J. Rowley (NHS
    funded)
Mrs J. Horsely (Dept.
    funded)
Mrs M. Jopson (Dept.
    funded)

Senior Technicians:

Mrs L. Harker (BHF funded)
Mrs S. Jamieson (BHF funded)
Mr P. Harrison (BHF funded-Project Grant)

Associated NHS Staff:
Mr C. J. Hilton (Surgery)
Dr A. Murray (Medical Physics)
Dr C. Griffiths (Medical Physics)
Mr M. McGuire (Medical Physics)
Dr T. Ashcroft (Pathology)
Prof. O. James (Medicine)

UNIVERSITY OF NEWCASTLE UPON TYNE

Freeman Hospital and
The Catherine Cookson Building of the New Medical School
1990

The Chair of Cardiology

Held by
Professor R. W. F. Campbell, MB ChB, FRCP

STAFF:

Senior Lecturers:
Dr S. S. Furniss
(BHF funded)
Dr C. Wren
(Children's Heart Unit funded)

First Assistant:
Dr J. P. Bourke
(BHF funded)

Research Fellows:
Dr Colin Doig
(BHF funded)
Dr Daniel Higham
(BHF funded)
Dr Theodore Bishiniotis
(British Council funded)
Dr Kishore Nimkheader
(self-supporting)
Dr Andres Loaiza
(self-supporting)
Dr Khanchit Likittanasombat
(British Council funded)

Senior Technicians:
Mrs L. Harker (BHF funded

Clinical Lecturers:
Dr P. C. Adams
Dr H. H. Bain
Dr R. S. Bexton
Dr K. Evemy
Dr R. G. Gold
Dr A. S. Hunter
Dr J. M. McComb
Dr D. S. Reid
Dr D. O. Williams

Associated University Staff:
Dr G. Chester
(Comp/E.Eng)
Dr B. Sharif
(Comp/E.Eng)

Secretarial Staff:
Ms S. J. Murray
(BHF funded)
Ms J. Rowley
(NHS funded)
Mrs J. Horsely
(Dept. funded)
Mrs M. Jopson
(Dept. funded)

Mrs S. Jamieson (BHF funded)

Associated NHS Staff:
    Mr C. J. Hilton (Surgery)
    Dr A. Murray (Medical Physics)
    Dr C. Griffiths (Medical Physics)
    Mr M. McGuire (Medical Physics)
    Dr T. Ashcroft (Pathology)

Hons B.Med.Sci. Students:
    Mr Mark Kellett
    Mr Ian Nichol

UNIVERSITY OF
NEWCASTLE UPON TYNE

Freeman Hospital
1993

The Chair of Cardiology

Held by:
Professor R. W. F. Campbell BSc MB FRCP

STAFF

Senior Lecturers:
Dr S. S. Furniss (BHF funded)
Dr J. P. Bourke (BHF funded)

First Assistant:
Dr J. C. Doig (BHF funded)
(currently on BHF overseas fellowship funded)

Research Fellows:
Dr T. Gumbrielle (BHF/Dept. funded)
Dr A. Loaiza (self-supporting)
Dr Quan Fang (Brit. Council/Dept. funded)
Dr P. Kittipawong (self-supporting)
Dr K. Adalet (self-supporting)
Mr D. Thompson (BHF funded)
Mr R. Clayton (BHF funded)
Mr N. McLoughlin (BHF funded)
Dr M. Farrer (BHF funded)
Dr J. Skinner (Regional funding)
Dr A. Kamel (Egyptian Government)

Secretarial Staff:
Ms H. Dunn (BHF funded)
Ms C. Wigham (NHS funded)
Mrs S. Brougham (NHS funded)
Mrs J. Jopson (University funded)
Systems Manager:

Mrs S. Jamieson (BHF funded)

Hons B.Med.Sci. Students:
    Mr G. Thomas
    Mr R. Saharia

Associated University Staff:
    Dr B. Sharif (Comp/E.Eng)
    Dr G. Chester (Comp/E.Eng)
    Dr G. Rodrigo (Physiology Dept)

Associated NHS Staff and Clinical Lecturers
    Dr P. C. Adams (Cardiology)
    Dr T. Ashcroft (pathology)
    Dr H. H. Bain (Paediatric Cardiology)
    Dr J. Barker (Cardiology)
    Dr R. S. Bexton (Cardiology)
    Mr J. Dark (Cardiothoracic Surgery)
    Dr K. Evemy (Cardiology)
    Dr C. Griffiths (Medical Physics)
    Dr D. Higham (Cardiology)
    Mr C. J. Hilton (Cardiothoracic Surgery)
    Dr A. S. Hunter (Paediatric Cardiology)
    Dr M. H. Khalid (Cardiology)
    Dr R. J. Madar (Paediatric Cardiology)
    Dr J. M. McComb (Cardiology)
    Mr M. McGuire (Medical Physics)
    Dr A. Murray (Medical Physics)
    Dr J. O'Sullivan (Paediatric Cardiology)
    Dr G. Parry (Cardiology)
    Dr I. Purcell (Cardiology)
    Dr D. S. Reid (Cardiology)
    Dr D. O. Williams (Cardiology)
    Dr C. Wren (Paediatric Cardiology)
    Dr J. Wylie (Paediatric Cardiology)

UNIVERSITY OF NEWCASTLE UPON TYNE

Freeman Hospital
1995

The Chair of Cardiology

Held by:
Professor R. W. F. Campbell BSc MB FRCP

STAFF

Senior Lecturers:
    Dr S. S. Furniss (BHF funded)
    Dr J. P. Bourke (BHF funded)

First Assistant:
    Dr J. C. Doig (BHF funded until Sept. 1995)
    Dr P. Illes (BHF funded from Nov. 1995)

Systems Manager
    Mrs S. Jamieson (Dept. funded)

Research Fellows:
    Dr T. Gumbrielle (Dept. funded until Aug. 1995)
    Dr C. Plummer (Dept. funded)
    Dr E. Simeonidou (self support)
    Dr S. Roy (self support)
    Mr R. Clayton (BHF funded)
    Dr S. Karnchanapimai (Thai Govt. funded)
    Dr M. Farrer (BHF funded until Nov. 1994)
    Dr J Skinner (Regional funding until June 1995)
    Dr N. McLoughlin (BHF funded until Nov. 1995)

Secretarial Staff:
    Ms H. Dunn (BHF funded)
    Ms M. Carter (NHS funded)
    Ms C. Lawson (University funded)

Research Associates:
>Mr S. Yeats (Dept. funded)
>Ms J. Yallop (BHF Project funded)
>Mrs T. Donelly (BHF Project funded)

Hons B.Med.Sci. Student
>Miss A. Arya
>M.Phil. Postgraduate Student
>Dr Q. Fang (University Scholarship)

Associated NHS Staff and Clinical Lecturers
>Dr P. C. Adams (Cardiology)
>Dr T. Ashcroft (Pathology)
>Dr H. H. Bain (Paediatric Cardiology)
>Dr R. S. Bexton (Cardiology)
>Mr J. Dark (Cardiothoracic Surgery)
>Dr K. Evemy (Cardiology)
>Mr J. Forty (Cardiothoracic Surgery)
>Dr C. Griffiths (Medical Physics)
>Dr D. Higham (Cardiology)
>Mr C. J. Hilton (Cardiothoracic Surgery)
>Dr A. S. Hunter (Paediatric Cardiology)
>Dr R. J. Madar (Paediatric Cardiology)
>Dr J. M. McComb (Cardiology)
>Mr M. McGuire (Medical Physics)
>Dr A. Murray (Medical Physics)
>Dr G. Parry (Cardiology)
>Dr I. Purcell (Cardiology)
>Dr D. S. Reid (Cardiology)
>Dr D. O. Williams (Cardiology)
>Dr C. Wren (Paediatric Cardiology)
>Dr J. Wylie (Paediatric Cardiology)

MEMBERS OF
NEWCASTLE CARDIAC CLUB

Adams, P. C.	Physician-R.V.I.	Member 28.11.87
Bain, H. H.	Paediatrician-FH	Member 9.7.77
Barnsley, W. C.	Surgeon-S.B. and F.H.	Original Member 1949 retired 16.6.73
Bethune, M. B. (Farmer)	Paediatrician-S.B.	Temporary Member 12.10.57 Member 7.5.60 Retired 2.11.74
Behl, P. R.	Surgeon-F.H.	Member 9.7.88 Resigned 1992
Bexton, R. S.	Physician-F.H.	Member 19.10.85
Blesovsky, A.	Surgeon-S.B. & F.H.	Temporary Member 26.1.66 Member 4.2.67 Retired 1989
Bremer, C.	Physician-Sunderland	Member 22.4.51 Retired 10.3.73
Brown, A. H.	Surgeon-F.H.	Member 9.7.78
Cameron, S. M. (Hales)	Radiologist-N.G.H.	Temporary Member 15.10.60 Resigned 11.5.66
Campbell, R. W. F.	Physician-F. H.	Member –79
Dark, J. H.	Surgeon-F. H.	Member 17.7.87
Davidson, L. A. G.	Physician (SR)-R.V.I.	Temporary member 21.11.54 Resigned 4.2.56
Davidson, S. W.	Radiologist-R.V.I.	Original member 1949 'Retired' 26.1.66
Dewar, H. A.	Physician-R.V.I.	Original Member 1949 Retired 11.3.78
Dobson, R.	Surgeon-S.B. & Seaham	Temporary Member 9.2.63 Member 4.2.67 Retired 1980
Edmunds, A. W. B.	Physician-Darlington	Member 27.10.73 Resigned 10.10.81
Evemy, K. L.	Physician-N.G.H.	Member 19.3.83 Hon. Sec. 16.4.91 to 21.6.94
Farmer (see Bethune)		
Freeman, R.	Microbiologist	Member 10.10.81

Furniss, S. S.	Physician (Sen. Lect.)-F.H.	Member 31.3.90
Gold, R. G.	Physician-S.B. & F.H.	Member 21.10.67
		Retired 1992
Griffin, S. G.	Surgeon-S.B. & Seaham	Member 29.1.50
		Retired 11.3.78
Hales (see Cameron)		
Hall, R. J. C.	Physician-R.V.I.	Member 11.3.78
		Resigned 28.3.87
Henderson, C. B.	Physician-N.G.H. & S.B.	Temporary Member 11.7.54
		Member 7.5.60
		Hon. Sec 5.2.72 to 4.7.81
		Retired 4.7.81
Hilton, C. J.	Surgeon-F.H.	Member 23.2.80
		Hon. Sec. 4.7.86 to 16.4.91
Holden, M. P.	Surgeon-F.H.	Member 2.11.76
Hunter, A. S.	Paediatrician-F.H.	Member 29.6.74
Hume, W. E.	Physician-R.V.I.	Original Member 1949
		Last Meeting 15.2.58
		Died 1.1.60
Jackson, F. S.	Physician-N.G.H.	Member 12.11.50
		Retired 5.3.77
Julian, D. G.	Physician-F.H.	Member 2.11.74
		Resigned 1986
Mason, G. A.	Surgeon-S.B.	Original Member 1949
		Retired 11.5.66
McCuish, R. K.	Physician (S.R.)-S.B.	Temporary Member 28.4.56
		Resigned 15.2.58
McComb, J. M.	Physician-F.H.	Member 8.11.86
McGregor, C. G. A.	Surgeon-F.H.	Member 16.3.85
		Resigned 17.7.87
Mitchell, L.	Radiologist-F.H.	Member 31.3.90
Morritt, G. N.	Surgeon-F.H.	Member 19.3.83
Mowbray, R. M.	Physician-Dryburn	Original Member 1949
		(Hon. Sec. 22.4.51 to 5.2.72)
		Retired 24.2.78
Owen, S. G.	Physician (S.R.)-R.V.I.	Temporary Member 25.10.58
		Member 11.5.66
		Resigned 10.2.68
Pearson, D. T.	Anaesthetist-S.B. & F.H.	Member 23.11.68
Reid, D. S.	Physician-F.H.	Member 9.7.77
Summerling	M. D., Radiologist-F.H	.Member 9.7.77
		Retired 31.2.90
Swan, W. G. A.	Physician-N.G.H.	Original Member 1949
		Retired 16.6.73

Szekely, P.	Physician-N.G.H.	Original Member 1949 Retired 5.7.75
Terry, G.	Physician-Dryburn	Member 24.2.79
Tynan, M. J.	Paediatrician-F.H.	Member 5.2.72 Resigned 1977
Urquhart, W.	Radiologist-N.G.H.	Member 1965 Died 1979
Williams, A.	Physician- Middlesbrough	Temporary Member 15.10.60 Retired 7.3.81
Williams, D. O.	Physician-F.H.	Member 1.11.75 Hon. Sec. 4.7.81 to 12.7.86
Wren, C.	Paediatrician-F.H.	Member 25.2.89

MEETINGS OF THE NORTHERN
REGIONAL CARDIOLOGY GROUP

Date	Venue	Speaker	Subject
July 1981	Durham	D. G. Julian (Newcastle)	Secondary prevention following myocardial infarction
October 1981	Darlington	D. O. Williams (Newcastle)	Non-surgical techniques to revasciularize ischaemic myocardium
May 1982	Washington	R. W. F. Campbell (Newcastle)	The management of non-ischaemic cardiac arrhythmias
September 1982	Durham	R. Cory-Pearce (Papworth)	Cardiac transplantation
October 1982	Cumbria	D. J. Coltart (London)	Cardiac biopsy – is it necessary?
April 1983	Corbridge	R. Freeman (Newcastle)	Infective endocarditis
October 1983	Lancaster	A. L. Muir (Edinburgh)	Clinical aspects of nuclear cardiology
		J. B. Irving	After myocardial infarction
March 1984	Morpeth	R. J. C. Hall (Newcastle)	Thrombo-embolic disease
June 1984	Darlington	D. S. Reid (Newcastle)	Exercise testing
September 1984	Durham	Sir B. Barrett-Boyes (New Zealand)	Valve surgery – past, present and future
November 1984	Lancaster	C. Wilson (Belfast)	Mobility coronary care
		R. G. Charles (Liverpool)	Cardiac team – Groote-Schuur Hospital
March 1985	Darlington	G. Williams (Leeds)	Doppler echocardiography
July 1985	Newcastle	S. Hunter (Newcastle)	Non-surgical treatment of congenital heart disease

Date	Venue	Speaker	Subject
November 1985	Cumbria	Prof. J. Camm (London)	Diagnosis and management of arrhythmias – **Failed to appear**
		R. G. Gold (Newcastle)	Pacemakers of the future
February 1986	Durham	D. G. Julian (Newcastle)	Acute intervention following myocardial infarction (Professor Julian's farewell dinner)
June 1986	Northallerton	J. Taylor (Dept. of Transport)	Cardiological aspects of fitness to drive
October 1986	Cumbria	R. W. F. Campbell	Fits, faints and Funny turns. Cardiological causes
		N. E. F. Cartlidge	Neurological causes
		R. A. L. Brewis (Newcastle)	History of the Town Moor
June 1987	Hexham	J. McComb (Newcastle)	Electrophysiological Studies in the diagnosis and treatment of arrhythmias
October 1987	Cumbria	R. Freeman (Newcastle)	Myocarditis
		A. H. Brown	Results of CABG surgery
		A. Martin (Sunderland)	'Aperitif' from Sudan
July 1988	Teeside	P. Adams (Newcastle)	Thrombolytic therapy in myocardial infarction
October 1988	Cumbria	S. Hillis (Glasgow)	treatment of heart failure
		J. Dark (Newcastle)	The Future of Heart/Lung Transplantation
		R. Freeman (Newcastle)	Derivation of Words and Phrases
June 1989	Durham	C. Wren (Newcastle)	Arrhythmias in Children
October 1989	Cumbria	G. Davies (London)	Silent Ischaemia
		C. Day (Newcastle)	Q-T Interval
		H. A. Dewar (Newcastle)	History of Newcastle Cardiology

Date	Venue	Speaker	Subject
April 1990	Teesside [Wynyard Hall]	J. Dark (Newcastle)	Heart Lung Transplantation
June 1990	Teesside	M. Laker (Newcastle)	Lipid Screening
January 1991	Cumbria	J. M. McComb (Newcastle)	Supraventricular Arrhythmias (The windiest, wettest weekend in Lake District History!)
May 1991	Darlington	D. G. Julian (London)	The British Heart Foundation
November 1991	Cumbria	A. L. Muir (Edinburgh)	Advances in the Management of Heart Failure
		P. Nichols (Belfast)	Hyperlipidaemia
October 1992	Cumbria	R. Freeman (Newcastle)	Recent Advances in Infective Endocarditis
		C. Cowan (Leeds)	Atrial Fibrillation
		J. Winch Q.C.	Doctor in the Witness Box
October 1993	Cumbria	A. Kenny (Newcastle)	Echocardiography

APPENDIX V

GLOSSARY OF MEDICAL TERMS

Angiography. The injection into the blood-stream of a fluid which will show up on an X-ray and outline hollow structures.

Aneurysm. A pulsating collection of blood encased in clot, and still connected to the artery from which it escaped.

Arrhythmia. Loosely used for disturbed rhythm of the heart.

Asystole. The heart does not beat at all.

Atherosclerosis. Popularly known as hardening of the arteries.

Atrial Flutter. The atria beat very rapidly and regularly, but the ventricles only respond to a proportion of the beats.

Atrial Septal Defect (ASD). An abnormal 'hole' in the wall which separates the atria, (the preliminary pumping chambers).

Auricle. Strictly the ear-like part of an atrium, but often the word is used for the whole of it. Also called the atrial appendage.

Balloon Atrial Septostomy. A palliative procedure for an infant with transposition (qv) in which a small ASD is deliberately made by distending a small balloon at the end of a cardiac catheter.

Beta-adrenergic Blockade. Prevention of some of the actions of adrenalin.

Biopsy. A piece of tissue, taken from a live patient, usually for microscopic examination.

Bradycardia. Overslowing of the heart rate.

Bronchiectasis. an irreparable disease of a lung, which sometimes followed pneumonia.

Bronchogram. An X-ray picture of the bronchi, obtained by injecting a radio opaque fluid into them.

Bronchoscope. An instrument, enabling one to see the inside of the bronchi (the larger airtubes).

CABG. Coronary Artery Bypass Grafting.

Cardiac Output. The number of litres of blood pumped per minute by the heart.

Cardiographer. A technician, who records patients' electrocardiograms (ECGs)

Cardiomyopathy. Disease of the muscle of the heart.

Cardiopulmonary bypass. A mechanism, whereby a patient's blood is withdrawn through tubes into an oxygenator and then pumped back into the patient, so that temporarily neither lungs or heart are needed and operations on the latter can be performed without disturbance.

Coarctation. A constriction.

Coronary Sinus. The large vein through which the blood from the muscle of the heart returns to the right atrium.

Defibrillation. Terminating fibrillation with an electric shock.

Dissection. (most often of the aorta). Through a weak place in the lining blood penetrates to between the layers, separating them and blocking the branches.

Ductus (Arteriosus). A channel connecting the large arteries (Pulmonary and Aorta) which carry blood from the ventricles into the lungs and the whole body respectively. It is always present before birth, when the lungs are not working. It should close spontaneously very soon after birth, but occasionally remains open (patent).

Dysrhythmia. Disturbance of the regular beating of the heart.

Electrolyte. An element, such as sodium, potassium and lithium, which, dissolved in water, will enable it to conduct an electric current. In the body it can, in certain circumstances, pass in and out of a cell through its membrane.

Embolism. The carriage by the bloodstream of something, e.g. bubbles of air or a blood clot, from one site to another.

Empyema. A collection of pus between the two layers of the membrane (pleura), which encloses each lung.

Epicardial. On the outside of the heart.

Fibrillation. Rapid, irregular and ineffectual twitching of heart muscle.

Fibrinolysis. The dissolving of fibrin – the network which holds the cells of a blood clot (thrombus) together.

Haemodynamic. Involving the physical principles of blood flow.

Haemolysis. Destruction of red blood corpuscles in the bloodstream.

Heart Block. Impairment of the mechanism, whereby contraction of the ventricles follows that of the atria.

Hemiplegia. Paralysis of one side of the body.

Homograft. Grafting of tissue from a member of the same species.

Infarction. Death of a tissue, due to interruption of its blood supply.

Ischaemia. Shortage of blood to a tissue.

Lysis. The 'loosening' or dissolving of a blood clot.

Mitral Valve. The valve between the left atrium and the left ventricle. When open it has the shape of a bishop's mitre.

Myocarditis. Inflammation of the muscle of the heart.

Parameter. A measurable feature.

Pericardium. The two-layer membrane, in which the heart is enclosed.

Phonocardiogram. A graphic record of the sounds made by the heart, as it beats.

Pneumonectomy. Surgical removal of all or part of a lung.

Pneumothorax. A condition, in which air enters between the two layers of the membrane (the pleura), which encloses the lung, and causes the lung to collapse.

Prosthesis. A man-made substitute for a tissue e.g. heart valve.

Sinus Arrhythmia. A heart rate which varies with respiration. Anybody can induce it in themselves by deep breathing, but it is often present during normal breathing, especially in the young.

Stenosis. Narrowing.

Subendocardial. Under the inner lining of the heart.

Tachycardia. Rapid beating of the heart.

Tetralogy of Fallot. A congenital narrowing of the valve between the right ventricle and the pulmonary artery, combined with a VSD. The commonest type of 'blue baby'.

Thrombus. Strictly a clot, forming in arterial blood and composed mainly of platelets, but also used for any kind of clot.

Transposition of the great vessels. A congenital defect in which the aorta is attached to the right ventricle and the pulmonary artery to the left.

Valvotomy. When the cusps of a valve have, either as the result of congenital malformation or disease, become stuck together, so that they obstruct the flow of blood, the operation of separating them is called valvotomy.

Venae Cavae. the two large veins, which bring blood back into the right atrium of the heart.

Ventricular Septal Defect (VSD). An abnormal 'hole' in the wall separating the main pumping chambers.

Xenograft. The grafting of a tissue, e.g. a heart valve, from another species, such as a pig.

Index